# Cellulite
# solutions

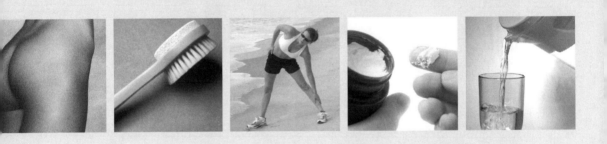

# Cellulite solutions

## 52 brilliant ideas
## for super smooth skin

Cherry Maslen & Linda Bird

**CAREFUL NOW**

We think we've managed to create a collection of ideas that will help you to improve your skin dramatically and make cellulite a thing of the past. However, while we love you and wish you every success in ditching the dimples we cannot take responsibility for how you choose to use this material. If you're planning to try out any home treatments please read the instructions carefully and consult your doctor or therapist before undertaking any therapies, taking supplements or changing your diet. In the end though, any decision is up to you and you are accountable for the consequences. It's your life, now get out there and live it.

First published in 2006 by
**The Infinite Ideas Company Limited**
36 St Giles
Oxford, OX1 3LD
United Kingdom
www.infideas.com

A CIP catalogue record for this book is available from the British Library

ISBN 1-904902-64-2

Brand and product names are trademarks or registered trademarks of their respective owners.

Designed and typeset by Baseline Arts Ltd, Oxford
**Printed by TJ International, Cornwall**

# Brilliant ideas

# Brilliant features

**Each chapter of this book is designed to provide you with an inspirational idea that you can read quickly and put into practice straight away.**

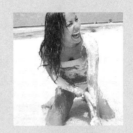

Throughout you'll find four features that will help you get right to the heart of the idea:

- *Here's an idea for you* Take it on board and give it a go – right here, right now. Get an idea of how well you're doing so far.

- *Try another idea* If this idea looks like a life-changer then there's no time to lose. *Try another idea* will point you straight to a related tip to enhance and expand on the first.

- *Defining idea* Words of wisdom from masters and mistresses of the art, plus some interesting hangers-on.

- *How did it go?* If at first you do succeed, try to hide your amazement. If, on the other hand, you don't, then this is where you'll find a Q and A that highlights common problems and how to get over them.

# Introduction

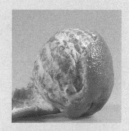

Chances are this isn't the first book on cellulite that you've picked up. But we're hoping it'll be the last.

Perhaps you've been struggling with cellulite for years. Perhaps you've tried every lotion, potion, diet or wonder-supplement going. And have yet to see results.

Or perhaps you've just been ignoring those podgy, pudgy, orange-peely dimples creeping down your thighs. Maybe you're resigned to it, believing it's part of a woman's lot.

It is, kind of. And at least we're all in it together. Between 85 and 95 per cent of women are plagued with cellulite, depending on whose statistics you choose to believe. It's as common in women as it is uncommon in men, which adds credence to that old adage 'it's a man's world'.

During our years at women's magazines we've encountered (and tried) just about every cellulite-busting diet, contraption and unguent money can buy. We've also met countless women – young, not-so-young, skinny or voluptuous, who are united in their longing to escape from Crinkly Bottom.

And the fact that nearly all women over twenty, even supermodels and A-list Hollywood celebs (if those paparazzi shots are anything to go by), are carrying cellulite somewhere on their bodies is little comfort. A dimply bottom, or thighs that take on an unsightly cottage cheese texture when you cross your legs, makes you feel blobby, unattractive, overweight, out of shape – and lacking in confidence. It shouldn't, but it does.

For years cellulite has confounded skin experts and beauty gurus. Is it fat? Is it caused by 'toxins'? Is stress a factor? Is it hormonal? With so many theories on what causes it, there's little wonder we've all been confused about how to get rid of it. We've written this book in an attempt to answer the questions and find some lasting solutions.

According to the leading dermatologists, fitness experts, fashion gurus, beauty experts and nutritionists we've spoken to in researching this book, the real culprits include being overweight, having a sedentary lifestyle and a bad diet. And, yes, lifestyle factors such as smoking, stress, and frying yourself in the sun all contribute. Beating cellulite, then, or at least reducing it, involves losing excess weight, taking more exercise, overhauling your eating habits – more green stuff, less fatty, salty and sugary stuff, and generally cleaning up your lifestyle.

But don't throw out all those expensive beauty creams yet. Some of them have been found to play a significant part in reducing cellulite. Salon treatments can help too. Plus, for those on a budget, there are a few effective at-home beauty regimes worth trying.

And for those (like us) who are impatient for results, we've also included information about some rather ingenious garments, make-up tricks and assorted tips that help disguise the problem. There are even some specially formulated undies that should be in every woman's lingerie drawer.

The bad news is we haven't found a miracle cure to iron out the dimples (and erase the years) instantly. But we have uncovered some clever, inexpensive and simple changes that can knock your bottom into better shape in a matter of weeks. Combine these with some inspired fashion-camouflage and a few savvy body-confidence tricks and you'll see your bottom and thighs in a whole new light. Who knows, you might even learn to love them...

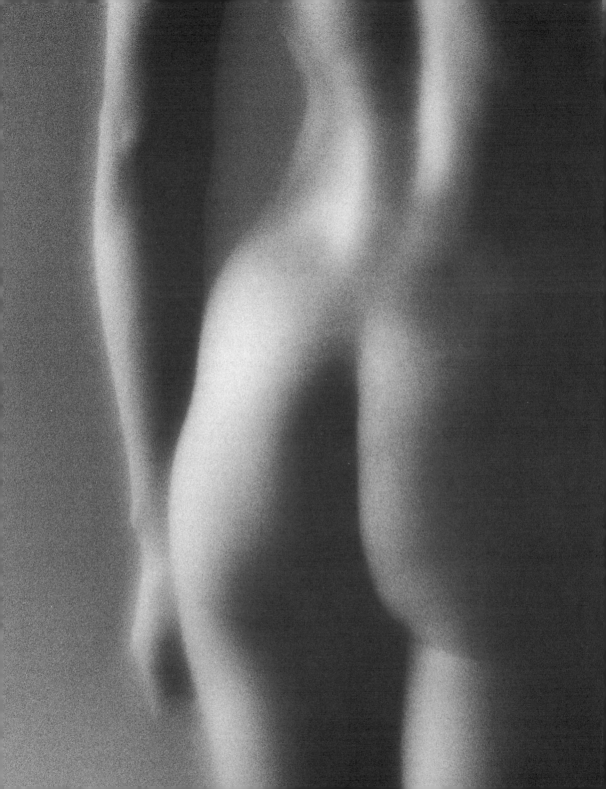

# 1

# Bottom's Up

**Celebrate your curves. Having cellulite – as nearly nine out of ten women do – doesn't mean you can't feel gorgeous. Try some bottom pampering today.**

The word cellulite was first coined back in the 70s, but it's no modern affliction.

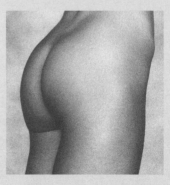

Just think of those Rubenesque lovelies, writhing about in the altogether. They'd never make the cover of today's *Vogue*, yet in their era they were considered the epitome of voluptuous sexiness.

Fashion has changed, and back in the days of yore, fatness (for that's essentially what cellulite is – body fat) would have been synonymous with wealth. Nowadays the smaller your thighs, the bigger your wallet. Women dread surplus pounds, aspiring instead to a neat peachy behind and racehorse legs. And cellulite, which becomes worse as you get older, is viewed as a sort of degenerative disease.

Face it. You know the horror you feel when you cross your legs and the orange peel bulges out. It's like viewing your first wrinkle or stretch mark. Somehow it's the beginning of the end.

The truth is cellulite is just part of being a woman – 85–95% of us fall prey to it, including the world's most glamorous models and actresses.

There's nothing disease-like about it either: it's surplus fat held together by skin cells that have lost their elasticity. And it lurks about the areas of a woman's body that are designed to lay down fat – backs of thighs, bottoms, tummies, even your upper arms. The result? Fat cells squishing upwards against your skin and causing a cottage cheese effect – like stuffing bursting out of an old cushion.

*Here's an idea for you...*

**Toning up your behind doesn't have to be a full-time occupation. Try this tiny bum-firming move which you can do anywhere. Raise one foot off the floor and kick it back behind you in tiny pulse-moves. Aim for 15 repetitions two or three times a day.**

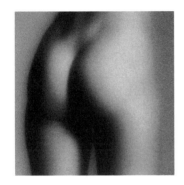

That's not to say you have to embrace cellulite as part of your femaleness (that's why we've written this book, after all). But before you get stressed, depressed and obsessed about the cellulitey bits, take a moment here to get a perspective, and to celebrate your curves.

A friend's husband once took a mould of her behind, which was, refreshingly, generously proportioned. He gave it to her as an anniversary present – a wonderful pumpkin of a bottom cast in bronze.

So the first lesson is 'remember, men love curves'. In fact men particularly love fleshy bottoms when they're paired with a small waist; studies show a waist/hip ratio of 0.7 is the magic formula most likely to get a man's pulse racing.

Don't forget too that your curves are there for a reason: making babies, having babies, feeding babies, filling out bikinis/ridiculously expensive undies, that sort of thing.

Your curves also give *you* pleasure. Legs, bottoms, thighs, tummies – they're all part of your healthy, functioning, living, breathing body. So think of a slightly dimply bottom as a sign of a rich, happy and fulfilling life.

Oh, and a spongy bottom is also handy at weddings and on bikes; pews and saddles can be so uncomfortable.

> Defining idea...
> **'Everything has its beauty, but not everyone sees it.'**
> CONFUCIUS

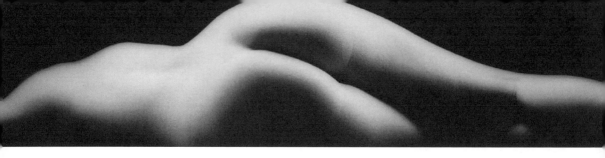

**So let's start by nipping that self-criticism in the bud. Time, instead, to celebrate that ass. Try some of these today:**

■ Savour the good things about your bum and thighs – the excitement of slipping into new silky pants, that satisfying pain/exhilaration when you cycle up a hill, the sensation of rubbing lovely cream into your legs, someone else fondling your behind...

■ Every day, promise yourself you'll do something that makes you feel good about your body – have something really delicious to eat, treat yourself to a day at a spa, go for a swim, book a fantastic holiday. Doing something pleasurable can make you feel happy.

■ Stop buying clothes that don't fit but which you're aiming to 'diet into'. They make you feel worse about your body. Instead, buy yourself something big but gorgeous that you can wear *now*.

*Try another idea...*

**Desperate (and rich) enough to consider surgery? Liposuction may appeal to non-squeamish cellulite sufferers who find diet and exercise a tall order. Read more in IDEA 38, *Suck it and see.***

4

■ Make a mental list of your best bits – hair, feet, long, beautifully shaped fingernails, trim calves, firm boobs. Stop focusing on your shortcomings and acknowledge your glories.

■ Splash out on body treats: indulging really does boost your self-confidence – book a facial/manicure, buy new perfume, wallow in a luxurious, gorgeous smelling bath. Take pleasure in looking your best.

■ Start taking some exercise. It can boost your mood, improve your complexion, help you focus and give you confidence in your body.

## How did it go?

**Q: I'm bombarded with billboards featuring images of teenage girls with super-smooth bottoms. How can I possibly feel good about my own bum?**

A: Invest in a beautiful coffee-table art book and peruse the images of real women that artists over the centuries have deemed beautiful – you'll find curves aplenty there. Visit galleries, muse over a Rodin sculpture. And think about your most attractive friends and colleagues. Do they have buttocks you could crack nuts with? Probably not. More likely they're confident, and exude *joie de vivre*. Remember there's more to beauty than the size and texture of your ass.

**Q: That's all very well, but what about all those holiday snaps of me looking round and dimply? Not very good for my body image.**

A: OK, so have a clearout. It's good therapy to get rid of old 'fat' photographs of you, which make you miserable. Instead collect pictures of yourself looking your best/slimmest/prettiest/happiest. It helps you realise you're a lot tastier than you give yourself credit for.

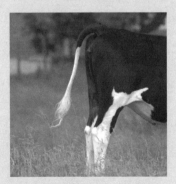

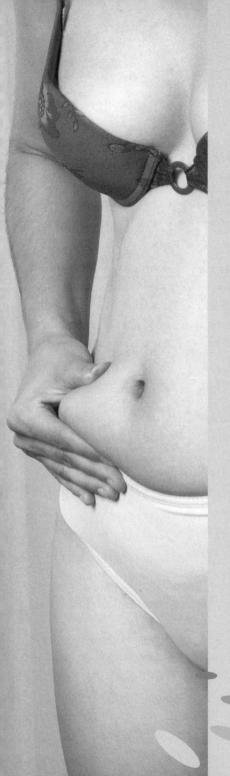

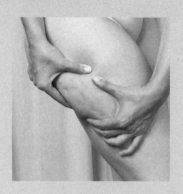

## 2

# Want to know a secret?

**Cellulite is fat – there's no getting round this. So drop some pounds and you'll shift some cellulite. Try our weight loss tips.**

Oh, if we had a penny for every column inch devoted to that mischievous demon cellulite, we'd be zillionaires. Orange-peely dimples are not some mysterious skin condition or bizarre freak of biology. Experts around the globe are pretty unanimous about one thing: cellulite is fat.

Simple as that.

More specifically, it's actually the top layer of fat, just beneath your skin, known as subcutaneous fat. When scientists conducted tests on the dimpled skin we get on our bottoms, tummy and thighs, they discovered that it was exactly the same kind of fat as that found on the rest of our body.

However, there's a reason why it looks different from the skin on the rest of your body. It comes down to the tissue that connects the fat to your skin and keeps it in place. This tissue is made from collagen fibres known as septae, which, in women, run in a kind of criss-cross fashion like honeycomb.

### So far, so straightforward.

But when a woman gains weight, the fat cells swell, and the fat effectively bulges out between the fibres. Imagine what a sausage looks like as it bursts out of its skin, or how stuffing can bulge out of an old mattress and you get an idea of what happens in your thighs and bottom. When the fat bulges out between the fibres, the result is those dome-shaped dimples we know as cellulite.

The reason why we get it on our bottoms and thighs is because when women gain weight, Mother Nature ensures the extra fat goes on our thighs, bum and tum as all those pear-shaped women out there will testify. What's more, even women who are slim elsewhere can be afflicted by cellulite, thanks to the distribution of fat.

> *Here's an idea for you...*
>
> **Want quick results? Try brushing shimmery bronzer on the backs of legs or thighs or smother thighs with a light-reflecting cream or lotion. They catch the light, making legs look smoother, and draw attention away from your cellulitey bits.**

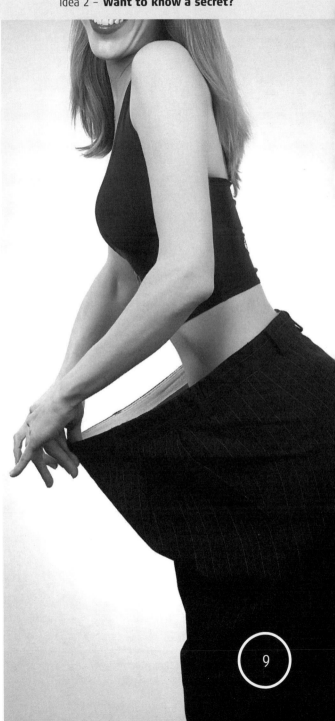

Try another idea...

**Ever seen a ballet dancer with cellulite? Dancing is a great way to keep slim and tone thighs. Pick up some easy moves in IDEA 46, *Dance with a stranger*.**

Fortunately, getting down to your ideal weight through diet and exercise means you'll shed some of the fat that causes cellulite.

Start by taking a long hard look at yourself. Could you shed a few pounds? Chances are, the answer is yes. Nearly half of us are overweight. Your medical practitioner, your gym instructor or a (brutally honest) friend can also help assess your weight.

Or try working out your body mass index (BMI). Your BMI is basically your weight in kilograms divided by your height in metres squared. So if you are 10 stone 4 lb (65 kg) and 5 ft 4 in (1.62 m), your BMI is just under 25: $65 \div (1.62 \times 1.62) = 24.8$

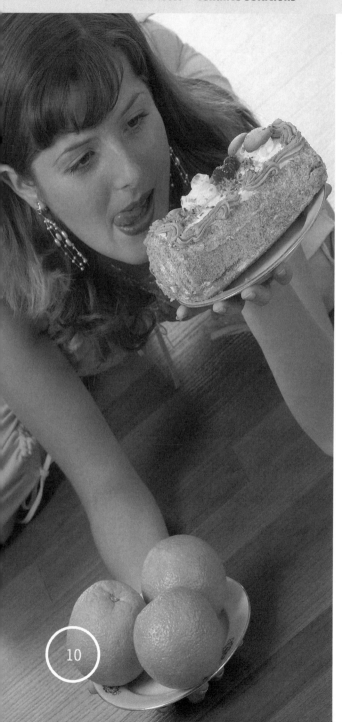

You can check out your BMI according to the following ranges, as used by the World Health Organisation:

| | |
|---|---|
| Less than 18.5 | underweight |
| 18.5–24.9 | healthy weight |
| 25–29.9 | overweight |
| 30–34.9 | obese |
| 35–39.9 | very obese |
| 40 or more | extremely obese |

If your BMI is more than 25, it's time to shift some fat.

Start small. Make some changes to your diet, such as cutting down on your fat intake, and swap processed, refined carbs – such as white bread and cakes – for wholegrains. Start taking gentle exercise: aim for 30 minutes of aerobic exercise at least three times a week. Brisk walking is a good place to start.

Try these five golden rules today to kickstart your weight loss:

■ Eat breakfast – as long as it's not a fatty fry up. Experts have found that dieters who eat a high-fibre breakfast lose more weight than dieters who skip breakfast.

■ Make sure you get your five portions of fruit and veg a day. Make them a priority before you eat anything else – you'll feel fuller already and will get more nutrients into your diet.

■ Never say never to treats. Depriving yourself of your favourite foods often makes you want to rebel – and you can end up bingeing. Instead, just have a tiny amount and use a teaspoon instead of a dessert spoon. Learn to savour instead of scoff.

■ Eat snacks. Yes, honestly! Eating healthy snacks – fruit, pitta breads and hummous, nuts and yoghurt helps keep your blood sugar levels steady – you'll never get hungry, so will be less likely to reach for cakes and chocolate. Aim to eat a low-fat snack every two hours.

■ Watch your portions: some people swear they eat healthily yet never lose weight. Huge portions may be the problem. You should be aiming for no more than a fistful of carbs and protein at one meal. But fill up with plenty of veggies.

# How did it go?

### Q: Why don't men get cellulite?

A: Because men's skin is thicker so their subcutaneous fat is less noticeable. Also, men's connective fibres, which hold the fat in place, are different – theirs run diagonally, so effectively hold the fat down better. Plus they're less prone to getting fat than us, thanks to the male hormone testosterone, and when they do it's around the tum rather than the bottom and thighs.

### Q: So cellulite is a hormone thing, is it?

A: Kind of. Female hormones are responsible for the distribution of fat over our bottom, thighs and tummy. Oestrogen also encourages fluid retention, which causes women's fat cells to bulge out more. Some women find that their cellulite gets worse when they're taking the contraceptive pill, or during or after pregnancy because their hormone levels surge. The more body fat you have, the more oestrogen you produce, so it's a vicious circle. But watching your weight can help.

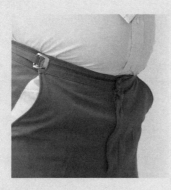

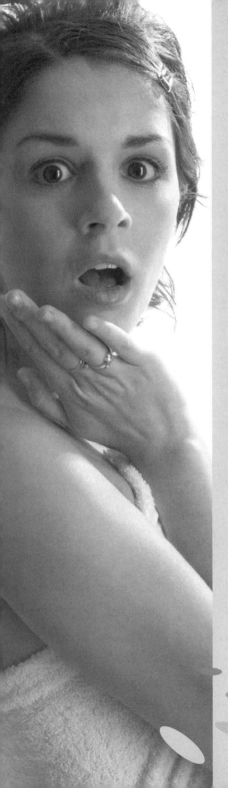

# 3

# Shock treatment

**Ionithermie's a no-nonsense salon therapy that involves sending rhythmic electrical pulses through your bottom. It might sound like a form of torture, but some swear by it.**

How do you like your massage? Administered by a dainty, nimble-fingered therapist? Or strong and firm and a bit on the rough side, with a muscley masseur to match?

Or how about the somewhat bizarre sounding four- or even six-handed massages that are all the rage these days – administered by a busload of masseurs at the same time?

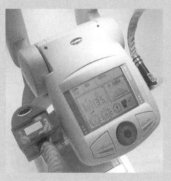

Then there's the machine approach favoured by those who need a firmer grip – some pull and pummel your body bits and do the job of about thirty therapists or more (without once asking where you're going on your holidays!)

Massage figures heavily in most anti-cellulite programmes because it's thought to help boost a sluggish circulation and lymphatic drainage, which may help skin texture and reduce water retention. The kind of unguents and oils actually massaged into the skin make a difference too; aromatherapy oils, marine extracts and clays all have active ingredients that go to work on circulation and skin cells, even burn fat or help boost collagen production.

One salon beauty treatment that comes, not surprisingly, from France combines both of these elements – massage and active products – and involves a machine to help the ingredients penetrate more deeply into the skin.

Here's an idea
for you...
**Sedentary lifestyle? Make a resolution: do some kind of exercise every day. It's good for your skin, your circulation and burns fat. Studies have shown that people who raise their heartbeat during exercise more than three times a week have improved skin elasticity. Start small: take the stairs instead of the lift, park your car further from the shops, get off the bus a stop earlier.**

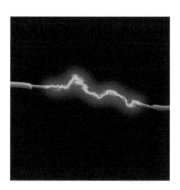

More specifically, ionithermie is a toning, firming body treatment that uses electrical charges – galvanic and isotonic currents – which are said to give the muscle a kind of friction-based 'workout', and thereby help firm up your buttocks/thighs too. Some say it's the ideal treatment for those people who have successfully shed weight yet still need help to tone and firm. Devotees say it helps with inch loss, and leaves your skin as smooth and silky as the proverbial baby's bottom (without the dimply bits).

Try another idea...
If you're waiting for a really quick fix to wobbly thighs, check out the technological advances just around the corner in IDEA 28, *Tomorrow's world.*

## What happens at a session?

You'll undress and the therapist may take measurements from your hips, thighs and bottom before she starts. You'll get a lovely body scrub, to exfoliate the dead skin cells on the surface, and then you'll be treated to a pressure point massage so you're relaxed and feeling better about life before the hard work on your bum really starts.

Then your cellulitey bits are covered with a thermal clay and essential oil-based goo sandwiched between layers of gauze. It's cooling and smells delicious.

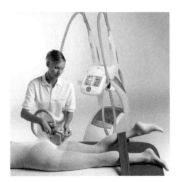

The warming mixture contains essential oils of cypress and pine which are thought to increase circulation, and work as a natural diuretic. These oils smell lovely and fresh and are known for their uplifting benefits (that's on your emotions, rather than your bottom, but you never know).

15

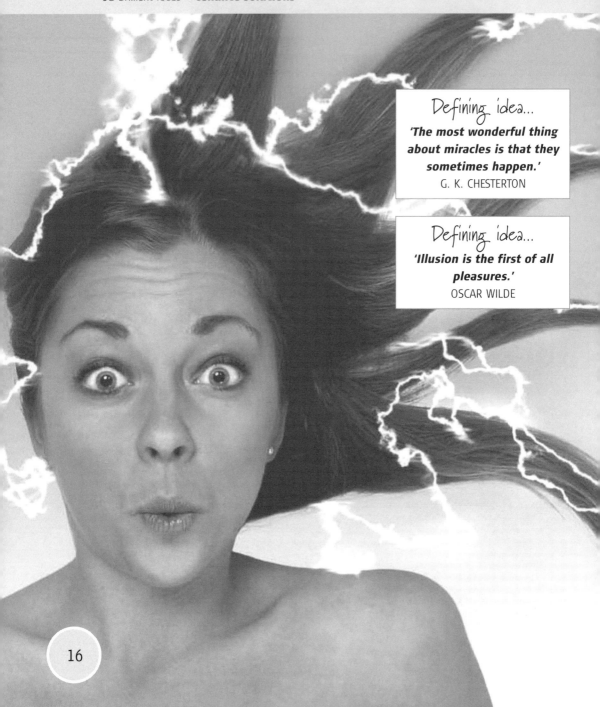

Defining idea...
'The most wonderful thing about miracles is that they sometimes happen.'
G. K. CHESTERTON

Defining idea...
'Illusion is the first of all pleasures.'
OSCAR WILDE

16

Then pads which emit rhythmic electrical pulses are placed on your skin. There's no need to brace yourself. You won't be bouncing off the bed or gritting your teeth to cope with the pain. The action is gentle – a combination of electrical stimuli that gets to work on the wobbly stuff, giving it a hefty dose of thermal clay and biologically active natural ingredients.

Defining idea...
'*Machines take me by surprise with great frequency.*'
ALAN TURING

When the pads are activated, the current pulses through your behind, and you'll feel the strange sensation of your muscles contracting while you lie there doing absolutely nothing. It's a strange, but not painful experience, and you can somehow feel it working.

They say that just one session of ionithermie is the equivalent of doing about 800 sit-ups! To relax you further, the therapist often gives you a lovely back massage, before taking all the pads and gauze and paste off your behind and removing the debris.

Expect to emerge with softer, smoother skin, and possibly looking a few inches smaller from behind, although don't bring your old jeans with you and expect to be able to slip into them. It's not that dramatic.

At the least it's a pleasurable experience, at best you'll lose inches, and you'll pay about £40–50 for the privilege. Experts usually recommend a course of five or six treatments, or more, depending, although results do tend to be short lived.

## How did it go?

### Q: Is there anything similar to ionithermie that'll work on the rest of my body?

A: Yes, there's also an ionithermie treatment to firm your bust. It usually takes about 90 minutes (be prepared to be topless for the entire process). In fact it targets all the floppy bits in your upper half. It's designed to lift saggy boobs and improve slack arms, and even claims to help you lose inches from your midriff.

### Q: What is the evidence that ionithermie actually works? Are there any impressive results?

A: Some trials have shown that ionithermie may help reduce your thighs by up to 8 cm in just one session. Independent studies have shown about ten treatments can improve orange-peely skin. In one independent trial, one woman lost 15 cm from her thighs after six weeks from ionithermie alone. But ideally, the best way to combat cellulite is with a three-pronged attack: combine healthy eating with regular exercise, and *then* treat yourself to beauty/salon treatments.

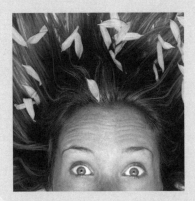

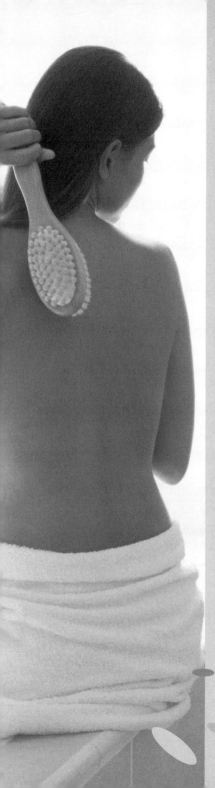

# 4

# Give it the brush-off

**Here's a cheap and cheerful solution to your cellulite woes. Daily skin brushing can help soften and smooth out orange-peel thighs. And you'll soon see the results.**

You'd be forgiven for thinking that you need a vast budget, and a coterie of beauty therapists and personal trainers to really banish cellulite.

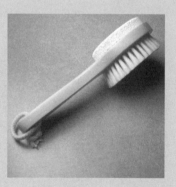

But judging by some of those paparazzi shots of celebrities and glamourpusses baring cellulite-stricken thighs, having lots of cash clearly doesn't guarantee you a svelte, smooth behind. In fact one of the most inexpensive ways to tackle a dimply bottom is to give it a good firm brushing.

Most beauty experts and authorities on cellulite agree that regular body brushing can dramatically enhance the texture of your skin and help the dimples appear less noticeable.

The advantages are you can do it every day in the comfort and privacy of your own home, that it takes no more than three to five minutes of your time, and that it costs nothing – well, a decent brush costs about the same as a bottle of wine. And that you can usually see results within days.

Body brushing can help minimise cellulite in two ways. Firstly, it helps remove surface dead cells, which makes the skin on your rear end look smoother and more even-textured. Think about how much smoother and more radiant your face looks after you've exfoliated; you get the same effect on your bum too!

Secondly, dry skin brushing is considered an effective way to stimulate circulation and boost lymphatic drainage – deficiences in both of these systems are believed to be major contributing factors to cellulite.

> *Here's an idea for you...*
> **Get the circulation in your bottom and thighs going, and smooth the skin at the same time, with a home-made scrub. Mix two tablespoons of finely ground oatmeal together with one tablespoon of almond oil. Rub into the skin, then rinse off in the shower.**

Ever noticed how blotchy and pasty your face looks when you've been sedentary or lolling about lazily for days on end in a centrally heated or air-conditioned room? Compare this to how it looks when you've taken some exercise, washed, exfoliated and patted your skin. Boosting your circulation improves skin dramatically.

*Try another idea...*
**Seawater is healing, refreshing, and can work wonders on a wobbly thigh. Check out thalassotherapy in IDEA 41, *Getting your sea legs.***

In fact many experts describe cellulite as a disorder of the lymphatic drainage system and your circulation. When these two body systems work optimally, your circulation delivers oxygen and important nutrients to your cells via blood, and the lymphatic drainage system removes the waste-products.

Think, then, of the healthy fatty tissues on your bottom and thighs. This tissue has a blood supply which provides nutrients and oxygen, and a drainage system taking waste-products away.

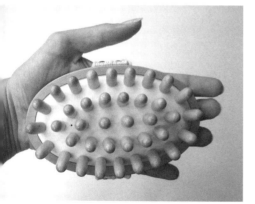

When this flow of fluid slows down, either because you live the life of a couch potato, or have a very sedentary job, your limbs don't get much action and your skin in that region suffers.

Your skin cells that separate the fat cells in your bottom and thighs are like bits of elastic. The more sedentary you are, the less nourished they become, and gradually they become thicker and less flexible. If you're a confirmed couch potato, the continued sluggish movement of fluid round your body makes these fibres even thicker and tougher.

And, because these fibres lose their elasticity, the fat that lies beneath them ends up bulging out between them, creating the dimples we know as cellulite.

All of this is made even worse by the excess fluid in the bottom and thigh area – which is another result of poor lymph flow and blood circulation.

Dry skin brushing, then, can help get your blood circulation and lymph flowing again. Plus some experts also believe that skin brushing helps encourage new skin cells to regenerate and boost collagen production, which in turn helps elasticity.

Convinced? Judge for yourself. Try it every day before your shower or bath and brush your skin in long strokes towards the heart.

# How to body-brush

Start at your feet and brush your soles, toes and ankles and top of each foot gently but firmly with long, sweeping movements. Brush the front and back of your lower legs, working towards your knees. Then rest your foot against the bath or a chair and brush from your knees to your upper legs and thighs, waist and buttocks using long, smooth strokes. Repeat on both legs.

## Defining idea...

'The buttocks are the most aesthetically pleasing part of the body because they are non-functional...as near as the human form can ever come to abstract art.'
KENNETH TYNAN, legendary theatre critic (and confirmed bottom-man)

Many women get cellulite on their upper arms, so don't neglect your upper body. Start at your wrist and brush your inner arm in upward strokes towards your elbow. Then brush the palm of your hand, then the outer side of your hand, and move up towards the back of your arm. Repeat on the other arm. Follow with gentle circular movements over your stomach and chest.

Then shower or jump in the bath to remove the dead surface cells.

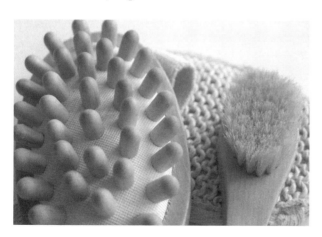

# How did it go?

### Q: Will a loofah be as effective as a skin brush?

A: Yes, choose either a loofah or a body brush with natural fibres – they're gentler than man-made fibres. Aim to do it every day before your shower or bath. The morning is a good time because it's invigorating and gets you revved up for your day. Then have a bath or shower to remove the dead skin cells. Wash your brush every few weeks with shampoo or warm water and leave it to dry.

### Q: Can I brush my skin when it's wet?

A: You won't remove the surface cells so effectively if your skin is wet, neither will your brush glide so easily across your skin. The key is to use long, smooth movements on dry skin towards the heart. Oh, and if you have a cellulitey tummy, brush that too, using very gentle circular movements – in a clockwise direction. Use very light pressure as this is a sensitive area.

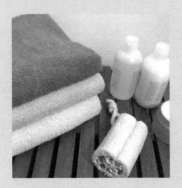

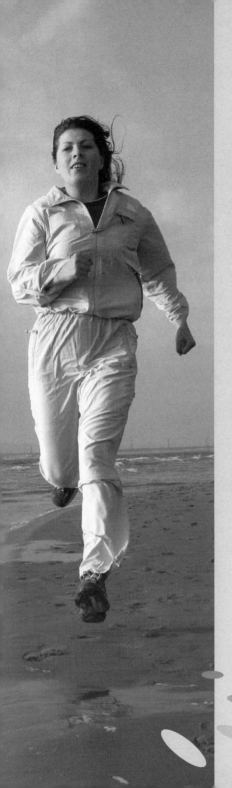

# 5

# Keep on running

**Jogging is one of the best forms of cellulite-busting exercise. Start small, aim high – even walking works wonders.**

Newsflash! You don't have to be sporty to fall in love with running. Just take it slowly and keep your goals realistic. Bear in mind that running aids weight loss, and is fantastic for toning legs.

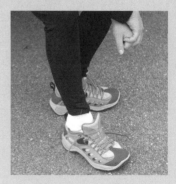

It's also a wonderful mood booster, releasing 'feel-good' endorphins that impart a lovely natural high. So if your cellulite gets you down, all the more reason to get running. In fact, research indicates that exercise may be more effective than antidepressants at treating mild to moderate depression. Little wonder it's so addictive.

Running is also great for your heart and overall cardiovascular health. It's good for your bones too: 30–40 minutes of weight bearing exercise three times a week can help prevent osteoporosis. Plus 30 minutes of physical activity three or more times a week can reduce your risk of breast cancer by 30%.

> Here's an idea for you...
>
> **Bin the biscuit tin, and instead snack on a big bowl of grapes. Grapes are rich in anthocyanins, which can aid collagen building – and having strong collagen will help reduce your cellulite.**

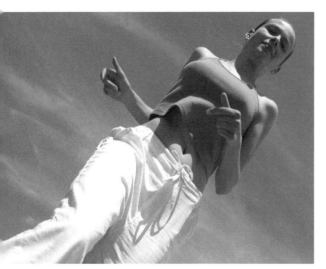

Because running targets your lower body, boosts circulation and helps burn fat and build muscle, cellulite doesn't stand a chance. Running burns a whopping 340 calories in 30 minutes. Plus exercising at a higher intensity, as you do when you run, kicks your metabolism up a gear even after you've finished your workout.

Running is a great way to shape up all over, really. One study showed that women who run more than 10 miles a week have smaller waists and narrower hips than women who don't exercise as intensely. Plus they also have lower blood pressure and higher levels of good cholesterol.

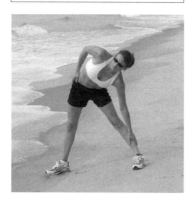

Try another idea...
**Need to make-over your eating habits? Perhaps a short-term detox diet could help. Turn to IDEA 45, *Waste disposal*.**

## How to start

Start small – keep your goals specific and realistic at first. But invest in great workout kit, a diary or notebook and water bottle. You're aiming to do about four workouts a week – but you'll be starting really gently. Always begin with 5 minutes of brisk walking and some stretches to warm up and prepare your body.

- Begin by walking regularly, for a couple of weeks or so if you haven't exercised for some time, then start to add short bouts of running to your workout.

- You're aiming to warm up for 5 minutes by walking, then run for say 30–60 seconds, then walk for 3 minutes. Then alternate the running and walking.

- If you start feeling breathless, switch back to walking again. Over a few weeks of workouts, gradually increase your running time and decrease your walking time.

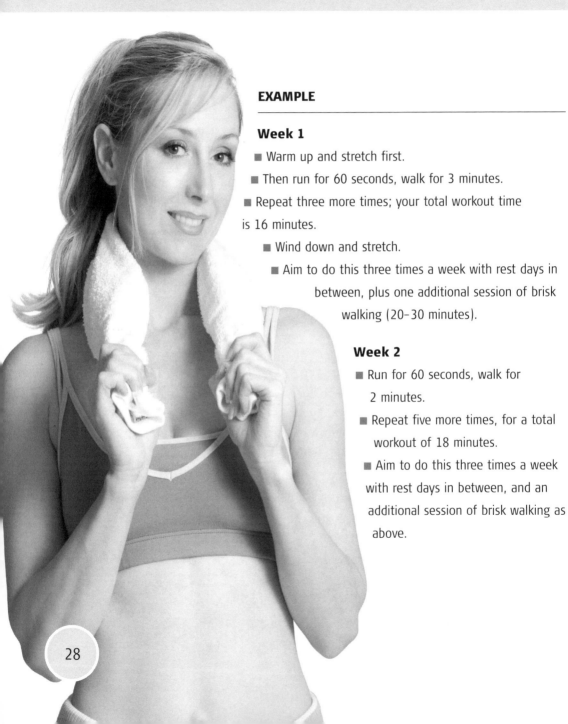

### EXAMPLE

### Week 1

- Warm up and stretch first.
- Then run for 60 seconds, walk for 3 minutes.
- Repeat three more times; your total workout time
is 16 minutes.
  - Wind down and stretch.
    - Aim to do this three times a week with rest days in between, plus one additional session of brisk walking (20–30 minutes).

### Week 2

- Run for 60 seconds, walk for 2 minutes.
- Repeat five more times, for a total workout of 18 minutes.
  - Aim to do this three times a week with rest days in between, and an additional session of brisk walking as above.

# How can I stay motivated?

- Write down all your reasons for wanting to get fit, lose weight, beat cellulite. Keep a diary of your progress, taking note of your weight and measurements before you begin your new running plan, how you feel after each session - and celebrating each tiny victory.

- Sign up for a race; set yourself a goal. Give yourself about 8 or 10 weeks to allow yourself time to get fit for it.

- Find a partner; research shows if you work out with someone else you're more likely to stick to it.

- Change your jogging routine - find a new route in the park or round your neighbourhood. And alternate your running days with a yoga session or aerobics/dance workout.

- Get outdoors. One Australian study showed that the natural endorphin high is greater for those exercising outdoors than indoors. Plus it means you get a good boost of vitamin D from sunlight, which is good for bones, teeth and cell growth. (Just be sure to wear sunscreen.)

> Defining idea...
> **'The only reason I would take up jogging is so that I could hear heavy breathing again.'**
> ERMA BOMBECK, humorist

29

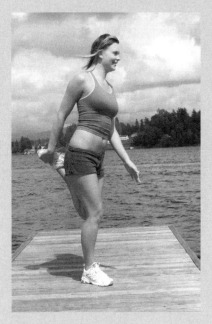

How did it go?

**Q: I hear lots of horror stories about jogging. Isn't it bad for you?**

A: Actually, running is better for your bones than walking slowly, as it's a high impact exercise. But it can put a strain on your joints if you don't wear the right shoes. Running shoes are designed to absorb the shock of pounding on the road, so make sure you find a specialist sports shop, get fitted and find the right pair for you. Also, seek softer surfaces, such as grass, running trails, or even treadmills. Oh, and invest in a really good, supportive sports bra with major bounce protection to avoid stretching your chest ligaments.

**Q: What's the best food to eat if I'm going to get serious about running?**

A: You need to eat for a steady supply of energy; choose carbs with protein or healthy fats. For a pre-run meal try a chicken, prawn, tuna or cheese sandwich on granary bread, or a jacket potato with baked beans or tuna, followed by yoghurt or a handful of dried fruit such as apricots. Also eat plenty of antioxidant rich fruit and veg to help mop up the free radicals that are released during intense exercise. Omega-3 fatty acids (found in oily fish and nuts) are anti-inflammatory and can help prevent injury.

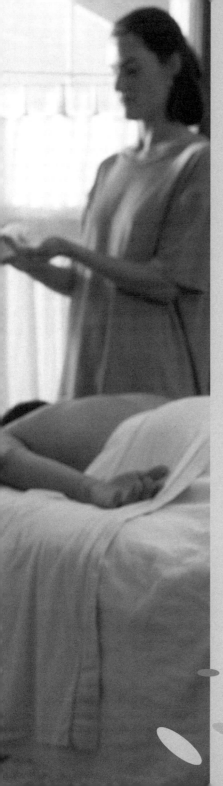

## 6

# Can you feel the force?

**Clinical trials have shown that endermologie, a deep massage therapy, can minimise lumps and bumps and reduce thighs by inches.**

You need some spare cash to take the salon route to cellulite-busting. But if you're rich — or frustrated — enough, one treatment in particular may reap rewards.

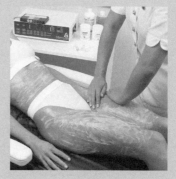

Have you stepped into a beauty salon recently? There's a massage, treatment, lotion, potion or therapy for just about every beauty challenge that afflicts us. There's no denying you emerge from a salon feeling buoyant, relaxed, slightly more gorgeous than when you went in. But with something as stubborn and prolific as cellulite, what kind of results can you expect in 45 minutes? It really depends how deep your pockets are.

Here's an idea
for you...
**Try cutting out that lunchtime cake and say no to that cappuccino. The money you'll save each week will go a long way towards paying for an endermologie session.**

Cellulite-busting miracles are hard to come by. That said, if you're serious about shifting cellulite, and are overhauling your eating habits, taking more exercise, and adopting all sorts of new bathtime rituals such as body brushing and self-massage, then a salon treatment can certainly yield positive results. At the very least, knowing that you're shelling out for a pricey beauty treatment may also keep you motivated and might help you remain more committed to cleaning up your lifestyle generally.

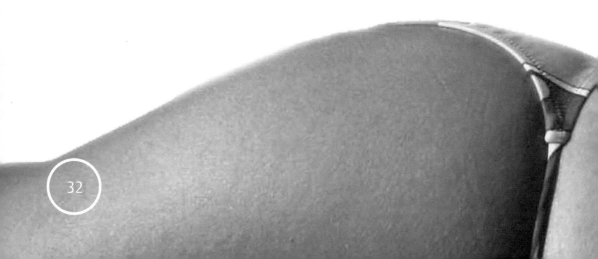

The key is to be realistic about your expectations. Most therapists concede that a one-off session isn't going to make a big, lasting difference; all treatments require a long-term course to show any real results. However, one in particular may help you turn a corner.

Try another idea...
**Has cellulite made you fall out of love with your body? Do you need a few reminders of why you're a gorgeous sensual woman – just as you are? If so, turn to IDEA 1, Bottom's up!**

Endermologie is a special form of deep tissue massage that uses a machine to stretch, stimulate, deep massage and smooth the contours of body fat, thereby reducing the circumference of the thighs or other areas of the body.

It was developed in the late 1970s in France to soften scar tissue and enable the skin to heal better. Researchers then went on to discover that using it to treat people for cosmetic purposes showed an improvement in skin texture and body contour.

Defining idea...
'**A beautiful woman and a wooden boat are very expensive in maintenance.**'
DUTCH PROVERB

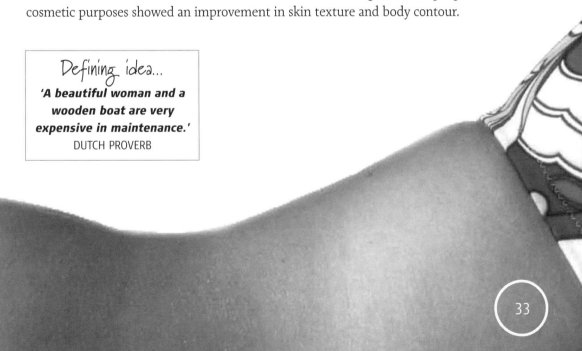

33

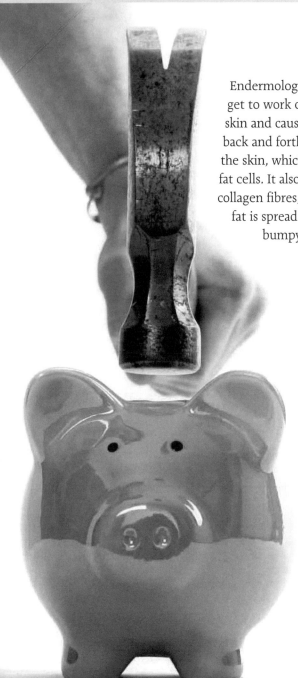

Endermologie is a machine-based treatment designed to get to work on the fat pockets that lie beneath the surface skin and cause you all those problems. As the machine rolls back and forth across the cellulite-ridden area, it sucks in the skin, which helps loosen and break down some of the fat cells. It also helps boost circulation, and stretch the collagen fibres, making them more elastic. Meanwhile, the fat is spread into a smooth layer, reducing the lumpy, bumpy appearance.

## What happens at a session?

Once you've undressed, the therapist helps you don a sort of elasticated body stocking (it's not a great look). Then, using a sort of hand-held machine, almost like a dustbuster-cum-iron, she massages the skin. Sounds painful doesn't it? Amazingly, it isn't. In fact given that the machine is giving your wobbly bits a thorough pummelling, endermologie is actually pleasant. The pain comes when it's time to pay! This 35 minutes or so could set you back about £70.

## Any good?

The good news is that, on paper at least, the results do seem impressive. In the USA, the Food and Drink Administration (FDA) approved endermologie as an effective temporary treatment for cellulite. It's one of only a few cellulite treatments with this kind of official endorsement.

In trials, it reduced the circumference of thighs and hips. One US study showed that after having seven treatments, patients lost about 1.34 cm from their thighs – and these *results were effective* even if the patients hadn't actually lost any weight. What's more, 31 patients who completed 14 sessions showed an even bigger average reduction of 1.83 cm.

*Defining idea...*
**'Patience, persistence and perspiration make an unbeatable combination for success.'**
NAPOLEON HILL, writer

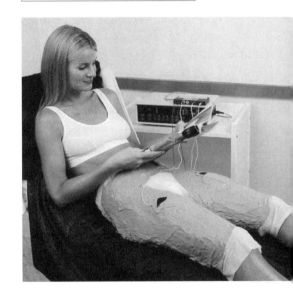

# How did it go?

**Q: So far so good, but does endermologie last?**
A: First, experts would agree that you really need to commit to about ten weekly sessions – or more, to see results. Thereafter you'd ideally need regular top-up sessions to maintain the results, so it's a big investment.

**Q: Am I right in thinking endermologie was originally used on horses?**
A: Apparently so – and have you ever seen a horse with cellulite? Quite. It was originally developed as a deep tissue massage in an equine unit for injured horses. It's also been used more recently to treat athletes. Results are impressive: it helps reduce post-workout muscle soreness, and improves their performance by 5%!

**Q: I can't afford endermologie. How can I appear thinner and more toned without dieting?**
A: Try this exercise every day, morning and night – within a week or two you'll notice a considerably firmer tummy, and narrower waist as it works on your core – the 'girdle' of muscles around your middle. Start off on your hands and knees. Position your hands directly in line with your shoulders and your knees in line with your hips. Tighten your abdominals and keep your back in a neutral position throughout. Now lift your right arm and left leg up in a straight line, then return to the start position and repeat with the left arm and the right leg. Try not to let either your shoulders or hips 'dip' whilst doing this exercise, i.e. try and keep as square as possible. Do two sets of 16 repetitions.

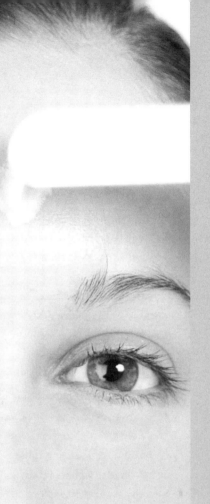

# 7

# Cream's crackers

**The number one beauty rule? Moisturise. Experts say keeping skin hydrated can help banish those dimples.**

'Moisturise daily' is the kind of advice dispensed by both your mother and beauty experts at glossy magazines. And while you know it can be great for your face, will it really help reduce cellulite on your bottom?

Skin specialists assure us it can. That's because when you slather on moisturiser, it helps plump out your skin.

37

The effects may be temporary but adding moisture can smooth out those dimples and orange-peel bits to a degree.

The truth is cellulite looks worse on dehydrated or dry skin. That's because when your skin lacks moisture, it looks thinner, so those little pockets of fatty cells beneath the skin (which are the cellulite) are more noticeable. If you rehydrate your skin, you reduce the appearance of cellulite.

Most of us don't need to be reminded to moisturise our faces, but the skin on the rest of our body often gets neglected. So aim to moisturise day and night – after a shower in the morning or after your bedtime bath.

Expensive, delicious smelling unguents make it a more pleasurable task, but any good moisturiser or body oil will do the trick.

Some of the best tried and tested brands of moisturisers include Dermalogica, Clarins, Decleor, and Nivea or Olay are great bargain buys. They make no claims about cellulite reduction, as they're simple body moisturisers, but with regular use, chances are your skin will look plumper and smoother and cellulite that bit less troublesome!

Moisturisers actually work by trapping the moisture into your skin (rather than adding moisture). But as you age, your skin thins and loses more moisture, so it's vital to use a

> ### Here's an idea for you...
>
> Add avocados to your shopping list. They're full of mono-unsaturated fats and vitamin E, which are good for your skin. They make a delicious snack. Chuck a few slices in a sandwich or over a salad. You can even make a moisturising beauty mask with them. Simply mush up two or three avocados into a soft paste and smother over your bottom – massaging it in using circular movements with the avocado stone (or get a willing bystander to do this for you!) Then just wash it off with warm water.

good cream or lotion as the years go by. Even petroleum jelly (Vaseline) works by trapping water into the skin, reducing water loss. And that doesn't cost an arm and a leg! That said, if splashing out on a pricey, beautifully packaged body moisturiser is going to make the entire process more pleasurable, then you may be more likely to build it into your regular toilette. And with moisturising, regularity is the key.

Another good tip to avoid dehydrating your skin is to avoid too hot water in your bath or shower as this can harm your body's lipids (natural fats). Don't soak for too long in hot water either. However sleepy or anxious you are to get between the sheets, make sure you do moisturise at night – experts say that's when the skin is more permeable so better able to absorb beneficial ingredients.

During dry weather or if you live in air-conditioned or centrally heated rooms, try using a humidifier to put moisture back into the air. Alternatively put a bowl of water on a radiator.

> *Try another idea...*
>
> **If you want the bronzed look without the drawback, check out IDEA 15, *Brown girl in the ring*, for self-tanning tips.**

Avoid over-using harsh soaps or detergent-based cleansers or bubble baths; these can strip the natural oils from your skin and make it drier. Experts say warm water is good enough to get your body clean – unless you're really grubby. Glycerine is a good ingredient to look for in soaps as this is really moisturising.

The sun is cruel to cellulite sufferers precisely because it conspires to dry out the skin, which makes those orange-peel dimples more noticeable.

When you lounge on your *chaise longue*, baking yourself in the sun, dangerous UV rays release nasty free radicals, which attack the collagen in your skin. This reduces its elasticity. On your face, this spells wrinkles. On your bottom and thighs it means

39

skin becomes more saggy, less firm and plump. The reason that cellulite gets worse with age is because the collagen and elastin in your skin become weaker and less elastic – and when they're less pliable, the fatty pockets beneath the skin aren't held in place and become more noticeable.

Best advice, then, is always to use a sunscreen (make sure it's at least a factor 15) and use plenty of it. Reapply it often and stay out of the sun between noon and 3 pm – the hottest part of the day. Better still, stick to fake tan, which is a great way to disguise cellulite.

Defining idea...

'I love to put on lotion. Sometimes I'll watch TV and go into a lotion trance for an hour. I try to find brands that don't taste bad in case anyone wants to taste me.'
ANGELINA JOLIE

How did it go?

**Q: Is it true that it's more beneficial to apply moisturiser onto damp skin?**
A: An old wives' tale, this one. The cream is actually diluted by the moisture on your skin, so you're effectively reducing the richness of the cream or lotion. Instead wait until you're properly dry before you slather it on.

**Q: What about exfoliators? Do they do any good?**
A: Again, there are temporary benefits. Exfoliating is a great way to brighten up the skin as it removes the dead surface skin cells, which can make skin look dull and lacklustre. When these surface skin cells are removed, the skin looks smoother instantly. When your skin is smooth, fake tan goes on more evenly – and we all know cellulite is less noticeable when your body's beautifully bronzed.

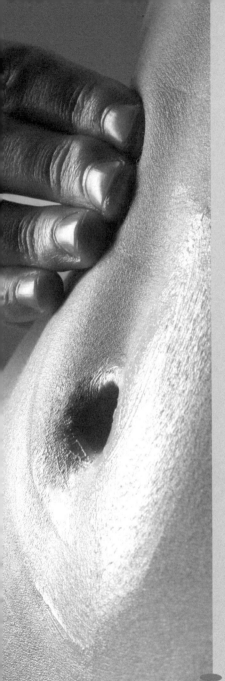

# 8

# On the shelf

**Cellulite creams abound. But what works, what doesn't and what's really worth the money?**

There's no denying the placebo effect of using cellulite creams — there's nothing like rubbing on pricey, sweet-smelling, beautifully packaged unguents to make you feel you're spoiling yourself.

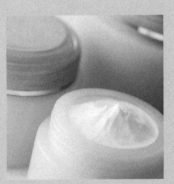

But, do they work? You might be seduced into thinking so. These days many products are impressively endorsed by various scientific studies, many of which claim that testers lost inches and pounds after using said unguent for a period of time.

But if you're hoping for a miracle in a bottle, you still have a long wait. Cellulite creams alone, however impressive, aren't likely to transform fleshy, saggy buttocks into a nectarine-firm bottom.

*Here's an idea for you...*

**Short on pennies? Try natural olive or grapeseed oil; you can buy them over the counter at chemists for next to nothing. Gentle enough for newborn babies, they're unlikely to cause reactions and are great for massage or for all over moisturising.**

But they may certainly help. Cellulite creams can hydrate your skin, so if your thighs and bottom have been neglected, rubbing on a cream will moisturise the area and help plump up the skin. Big difference already.

Many cellulite creams also contain temporary toning ingredients, which help improve skin texture; the effects can be pretty immediate but are temporary – good for a hot date, beach day, black dress occasion, that sort of thing.

But the longer-lasting effects come down to a pot-pourri of active ingredients, which do anything from boost metabolism, facilitate cell turnover, help shed water, even break down fat.

Take *caffeine*, a common and effective ingredient in many anti-cellulite formulations. It's thought to encourage the metabolism of fats, and help drain accumulated fluids in your fat cells, and boost your circulation. It's also toning.

Another key ingredient used in the more effective anti-cellulite creams is *retinol*. It's a derivative of vitamin A that has been found to increase skin renewal and boost the production of collagen. Often found in face cream, it can improve the elasticity of the skin on your nether regions too. RoC's retinol-based product has many devotees, who claim to have lost inches and firmed up significantly using the formulation twice daily.

Another cellulite-busting ingredient is *aminophylline*, which is thought by some experts to enter the bloodstream and actually break down fat in the cells. One study found women using aminophylline cream lost as much as 8 mm from their thighs. Another study showed impressive results with aminophylline, although it was used alongside a calorie-reduced diet and daily exercise too.

> Try another idea...
> **If you feel the need for something more than lotions, try microdermabrasion. It's a pricey salon treatment – a state-of-the-art version of exfoliation that helps reduce the dimples. IDEA 39, *Scraping the barrel*, gives the low down.**

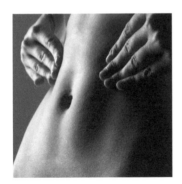

Exfoliating ingredients such as *alpha-hydroxy acids* (AHAs) are often used in the latest cellulite-busting products. AHAs are found in plants (citrus fruits and apples) and are used in skin products to help remove dead skin cells, thereby promoting the turnover of new cells. Thus far research has found that the effects on cellulitey areas tend to be temporary, rather than permanent, but watch this space.

# Natural ingredients

Most treatment creams are a combination of cutting-edge technology alongside tried and trusted natural or herbal ingredients. Here are a few to look out for:

- **Gingko biloba** can stimulate your circulation and boost blood flow. It's a strong antioxidant, so it may help slow down the ageing process and help fight the free radicals that can cause your skin to age.

- **Gotu kola**. This herb is thought to enhance the production of collagen. It's good for circulation and also has diuretic qualities. It's been found to help heal wounds and burns, so has positive effects on skin tissue.

- **Guarana** is a natural stimulant with a strong diuretic action. This seed is thought to help boost metabolism, and also has antioxidant qualities.

- **Horse chestnut** can help reduce water retention, boost circulation and increase blood flow to the skin.

- **Butcher's broom** is a plant extract with a diuretic action and may help boost circulation.

- **Ivy** has been found to help boost the circulation. It also has astringent properties, which may have a temporary toning effect on cellulite.

- **Marine extracts** such as carrageenan and alginic acid can help draw water into the skin, which may help make cellulite look less obvious by filling in the dimples.

- **Co-enzyme Q10** is a powerful antioxidant thought to help beat cellulite by helping build collagen, thereby countering skin sagginess.

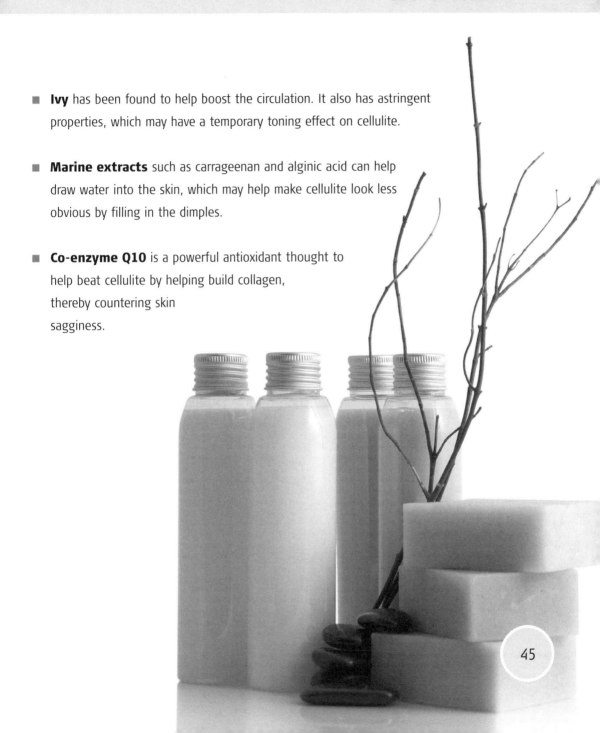

45

# How did it go?

**Q: I've been using this cream day and night for a week, but can't see any results yet. Am I doing it right?**

A: Have you read the packet? Many cellulite formulations are designed to be used alongside regular exercise and a low-fat healthy diet, and ideally applied twice daily using a five-minute self-massage technique, so the cream itself is just one prong in your attack. Most manufacturers also state the product needs to be used for at least 30 days before you see results. Also, bear in mind the results may be subtle rather than miraculous.

**Q: Are those massagers that come with the product any good?**

A: Depends. They're said to help you stimulate the area, and massage is believed to boost circulation and lymph drainage. Avoid rubbing over-zealously though; it can damage the tissue and make matters worse. Manipulating your cellulitey areas with a brush or loofah or special massager will certainly have an exfoliating effect, which can improve the texture of the skin instantly.

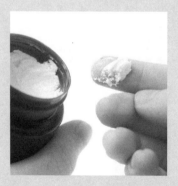

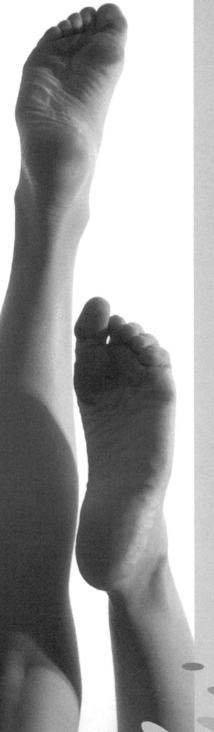

# 9

# The green goddess

**Here's the low-down on seaweed and algae body wraps. What really happens when you rub goo all over your legs and bottom?**

They don't call it the mysteries of the deep for nothing. If you've ever wondered why (on earth) women consider it a delicious beauty treat to smother themselves in questionable looking gunk and pay heavily for the privilege, it's time to wise up.

Body wraps have long been used as a cellulite treatment. The process goes something like this.

47

You go to a salon and undress, then a therapist applies some kind of blue, green or browny marine-based mud, then wraps your waist and bottom up in foil, or cling-film or some kind of gauze. Thus trussed, you're left gazing at the ceiling or floor for about an hour, after which you're cleaned, moisturised and sent out into the world, inches smaller and with smoother, firmer skin.

Seawater and sea products have been used therapeutically for aeons. Sea water is rich in important minerals – such as calcium, iodine, aluminium, magnesium, potassium, sulphur, zinc and selenium, which is a natural antioxidant.

These all have positive effects on the body – from rebalancing your metabolism and circulation, to relaxing your muscles, and also healing the skin, thanks to seawater's antiseptic properties. Seaweed and sea clay are also rich in iodine, which can help balance the thyroid function which helps regulate some hormone levels in the body.

Little wonder that people still flock to the Dead Sea with their aches and pains and for a beauty boost, and why you feel so fantastic after a dip in the ocean.

Marine products, then, are thought to help with cellulite by boosting circulation and encouraging fluid loss from the skin – so if you think your own cellulite is caused by water retention, it's worth investing in some of the green stuff.

The cling-film part of the process is thought to encourage the skin to sweat further,

> *Here's an idea for you...*
> **The sea has far-reaching benefits. Turn your dip in the sea into a cellulite-busting workout. Next time you're at the beach, try walking through waist-high water – this is great for toning the muscles in your legs.**

and you tend to lose water, which is why you often emerge having lost a few pounds and inches during the treatment. Sometimes the therapist will measure you before and after – any reduction in size does make you feel you've had your money's worth. Make sure you drink plenty of fluids after your treatment, though, as you could be dehydrated.

It's not a miracle solution, as the weight will return as you drink to replenish the lost fluids. But if you're bound for the beach, look upon it as a temporary cellulite-minimiser or tummy flattener. Plus it's actually fairly pleasant – deeply relaxing, and wonderfully pampering. And, appearance aside, the products usually smell delectable.

If your budget can't stretch to a salon treatment, you can DIY at home, bearing in mind that your bathroom will be mud-strewn and look like it's hosted the England rugby team post-match clean up (without any of the eye candy benefits for you!)

An altogether less messy route is to soak in a sea mineral bath – it's invigorating and leaves you with ultra-soft skin. Just lie back, relax and imagine you're a cellulite-free nymph swimming in the Indian Ocean. Great brands include thalgo (www.thalgo.com), Guam Sea Products or elemis (www.elemis.com).

Try another idea...

**Just had a baby? Looked at your thighs recently? Urgh! Those extra pounds during pregnancy can make your cellulite so much worse. Find out how to tackle it with some gentle postnatal care in IDEA 49, *Mums, tums and bums*.**

Defining idea...

**'Eternity begins and ends with the ocean's tides.'**
ANON.

# How did it go?

**Q: I've heard that eating seaweed is a bit of a beauty secret. Can it really work?**

A: Seaweed is a rich source of protein, low in fat and calories, which is good for your metabolism, and helps fill you up. So it's a great dish to choose if your cellulite is caused by excess weight. It's also rich in iodine, which is important for a healthy metabolism. Plus it's a good source of B vitamins, calcium and magnesium. Try getting more of it into your diet – look for arame, kombu, wakami and nori. Don't go mad though, and serve up seaweed for breakfast, lunch and tea; studies show that eating too much seaweed can adversely affect your thyroid.

**Q: What's that spirulina stuff I keep hearing about?**

A: Spirulina is another sea plant worth investigating. It's a green algae which comes in powder or tablet form and is rich in protein and minerals. It's known for its positive effects on cells, and is thought to be anti-ageing, so could be a good weapon in the fight against cellulite. It's one of the richest sources of calcium around.

**Q: What else can I do at the seaside to curb my cellulite?**

A: Learn a watersport: one hour of bodysurfing can burn about 177 calories; windsurfing about the same. Swimming's a great all-over exercise that can burn fat and calories, boost your skin tone and firm your wobbly bits at the same time. It has fantastic aerobic benefits, and is good for stomach muscles and a really effective way to build up arm muscles – useful if you have cellulitey batwings.

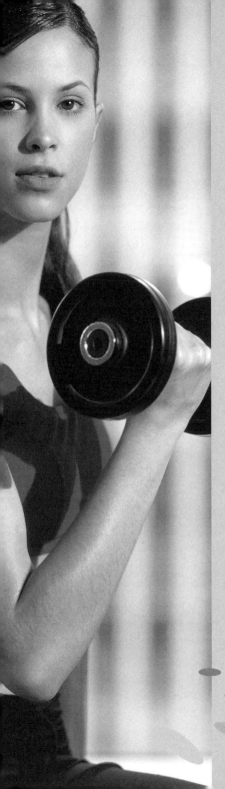

# 10

# I want muscles

**Muscle-building exercise can boost your metabolic rate and help you burn more body fat. Result: less cellulite.**

If you associate dumbbells with strapping lads in oversized belts, and think strength training is not something a delicate lady should contemplate, it's time to think again.

**Let's start with a few facts about muscles.**

The amount of muscle you have determines how many calories your body uses when you're inactive. Muscle burns more calories than fat (studies show just 500 g of muscle burns 30 calories a day just being there, whereas 500 g of fat burns just 2 calories a day!) So the more muscle you have, the more calories you burn.

*Here's an idea for you...*

Is water retention making your wobbly bits puffy? Try eating lots of natural diuretics such as celery, onion, parsley, aubergines, garlic and peppermint.

Regular weight training can increase your basal metabolic rate (BMR) by as much as 15%. (Your BMR is the rate at which your body burns calories – even just by sitting down, sleeping, breathing; the more muscle you have, the more calories you burn just by 'being'.) And you'll find you have bags more energy, too.

Then there are the bone-strengthening benefits of weight training. Some studies show that after six months of weight training, your spine bone mineral density could increase by 13%. Better bones help boost your posture, which helps make you look leaner. On top of that, regular weight training can help lower your blood pressure, fight diabetes and can improve your mood.

Lean muscle also fills out your skin, so saggy cellulite tissue could be transformed into neat, toned, smoother, taut buttocks in a matter of weeks. As you work on building and firming your muscles and reducing body fat, this effectively helps to lift the skin, which can help prevent that puckering which takes place when the fibres pull downwards. In fact, one study found that 70% of women said their cellulite improved in just six weeks by doing weight training on their legs.

The trouble with muscle is that when we reach our late thirties, we start losing it – about 250 g of muscle a year according to some figures. What that means is you risk losing 2.5 kg of muscle while gaining 7.5 kg of fat every ten years if you don't do anything to counter the muscle loss. So if you were to carry on eating the same amount of food and calories, you'd gain weight. Research shows that between the ages of 35 and 65 you gain about 500 g a year. Which is one reason why you may find your cellulite has become more noticeable over the years.

Try another idea...
**Did you know that certain trainers are made using special technology which helps bust cellulite? IDEA 40, *Getting a leg up*, describes the benefits of Masai Barefoot Technology trainers.**

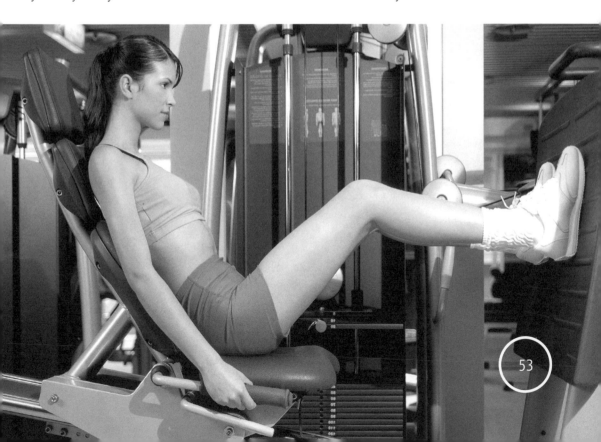

## What to do about it

> Defining idea...
> **'Muscles come and go; flab lasts.'**
> BILL VAUGHN, author

■ Get yourself a regular muscle-toning workout. Working with weight machines, dumbbells, barbells, body bars, body bands, wrist or ankle weights constitutes an effective resistance workout, so head for your local gym and ask a trainer to devise a workout for you. He or she will ensure you'll be doing things properly, so you'll be less vulnerable to injury.

■ The aim is to build in three sessions of resistance work a week.

■ Even using your own body weight as resistance counts, so you can even build your muscles at home; good exercises include sit-ups, press-ups, lunges and squats.

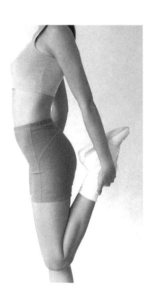

■ Turn your daily walk or cycle into an effective resistance workout by incorporating hills, or walking with ankle weights.

■ Gym-based classes such as step, spinning or body conditioning involve resistance work.

# What to eat for muscle power

- Cut back on fatty foods, and stick to low-fat meals, with plenty of fresh fruit and veg.

- Lean protein is important for muscles, as it helps repair the muscle fibres you may have damaged. So eat plenty of chicken, fish, tofu, lentils, nuts. Spread your protein evenly over five or six meals a day to maximise absorption and minimise fat gain.

- Calcium-rich foods such as dairy, beans and pulses help support healthy bones.

- If you're working out intensely in the gym, say three times a week, you'll need 1.4–1.8 g of protein per kg of your body weight. You also need carbs for fuel (bread, potatoes, pasta, noodles). If you're working out three times a week you need about 5–7 g of carbs per kg of body weight daily.

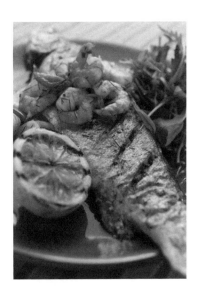

Defining idea...
**'Inward calm cannot be maintained unless physical strength is constantly and intelligently replenished.'**
BUDDHA

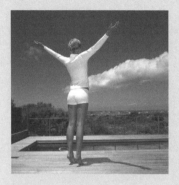

## How did it go?

**Q: The word 'muscle' worries me. Am I going to turn into a strapping Russian shot-putter if I follow this regime?**

A: Stop worrying. That's a common misconception. Fortunately, women's low levels of testosterone prevent them from turning into hulking great things. You'd have to take steroids for that. Or alter your eating habits significantly before you bulked up excessively. Supermodels and tiny Hollywood A-listers do strength training and even Marilyn Monroe used dumbbells!

**Q: Do I need to keep increasing the weights I'm using?**

A: Heavier weights don't necessarily mean better muscle toning. You'd do better to use lower weights but do more repetitions. However, you do need to exercise to near fatigue to really benefit from resistance training.

**Q: How do I do a lunge?**

A: Stand with your feet together holding dumbbells by your sides with your palms facing in. Take one step forward with your right leg. With your right foot on the floor slowly lower your left knee towards the floor, keeping your right knee at a 90 degree angle and your back straight. Press into your right foot and push yourself back to starting position. Repeat on the other leg. Aim for 12, building up to two or three sets over time.

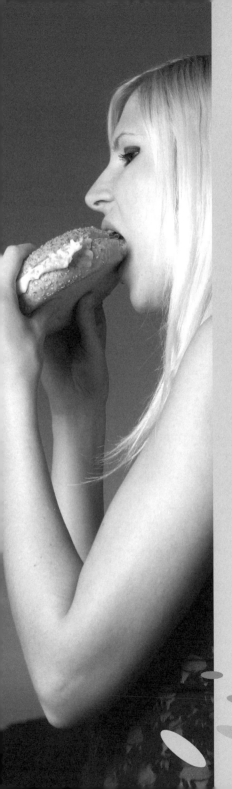

# 11

# Goodbye Mr Chips

**Cut back on fat and you'll reap rewards on your bum and thighs. Try some simple and painless ways to reduce fat in your diet.**

The trouble with creamy, fatty food is that it just tastes so darned good. But there comes a time in every woman's life when she has to choose between her bum and her tastebuds.

If you're reading this, no doubt your priority right now is on your behind. And, given that being overweight is a major factor in cellulite, it's time to slash some of the naughty stuff from your diet.

Let's start with some home truths about dietary fat:

**Weight for weight, fat contains twice as many calories as sugar.**
(1 g of fat contains 9 calories, while 1g of sugar contains about 3–4 cals) – so one of the best ways to cut back on calories is to reduce your fat intake.

**Fat calories make you fatter than carbohydrate and protein calories.**
That's because fat is closest to the form it needs to be for storage – to metabolise it requires just 3 calories for every 100 calories you eat. That leaves a whopping 97 to be stored in your fat cells.

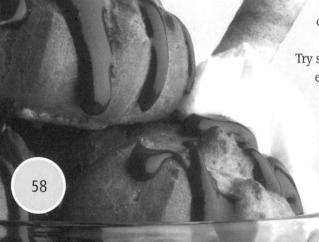

Compare this with the number of calories required to metabolise carbohydrates, about 10–15 calories which leaves only 85–90 to be stored. Protein wins hands down though; it requires an amazing 20 calories to use it. So if you want to boost your metabolism, stick to protein and carbs and go easy on the fat.

Try sticking to a moderate fat restriction eating plan (where it accounts for between 30 and 35% of your total calorie intake). You're much more likely to keep the weight off this way than with restrictions of up to 20–25% because it's more palatable and therefore easier to stick with.

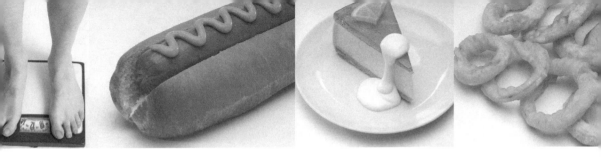

You don't have to suffer on a fat-free regime to lose weight. There are plenty of painless ways to cut back:

- **Ban** margarine, butter or cheese in your sandwiches (and use tuna, turkey and low fat ham as fillings). Mustard and low-fat dressings make good alternatives to spreads.

- **Reduce** red meat consumption by adding beans or root vegetables such as parsnips and turnips to casseroles or hotpots to bulk up your servings.

- **Keep away from** foods preserved in oil; check the labels and stick to brine or fresh water instead.

- **Stop frying food**; instead barbecue/griddle or grill your fish or meat.

- If you're making meat casserole, leave it to go cold, then **remove any fat** on the surface.

- **Never add** butter to your potatoes; try mustard or fromage frais in mashed potatoes instead.

- Drink clear broths or vegetable soups **instead of** creamy ones.

- **Never add cream** to pasta sauces or soups.

> Here's an idea for you...
>
> **Can't say no to afternoon tea? Try munching warmed fruit loaf with your cuppa instead of butter-laden crumpets; fruit loaf is rich in fibre and iron and is gooey and moist so you won't need oodles of butter.**

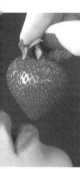

## Try these swaps:

- Instead of steamed puddings and cream, opt for crumbles; they'll keep your fruit intake high. Plus if you swap heavy crumble mixture for brown-breadcrumbs and a sprinkling of brown sugar you'll keep it lower calorie still. Serve with (reduced fat) custard and you'll get plenty of calcium.

## Try another idea...

If dieting, exercise, rubbing in lotions and potions to bust cellulite seems too much like hard work, think laterally. For tips on boudoir lighting and other ways to hide those dimples see IDEA 18, *Come to bed thighs.*

- Instead of toast smothered with butter – try hummous – it's a good source of protein, plus it's high in soluble fibre which lowers cholesterol levels.

- Love roasts? Swap red meat for white meat – and use spray olive oils and balsamic vinegar to add taste and cut back on fat.

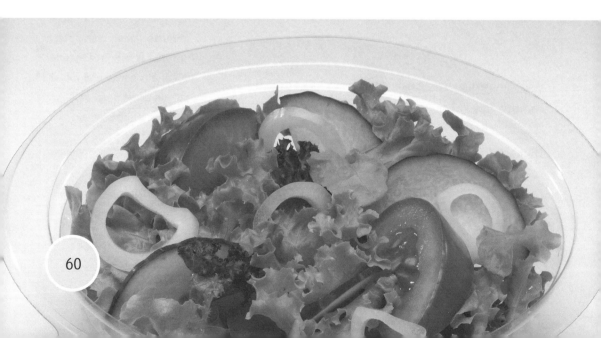

## Good fats

> Defining idea...
>
> ***'A fat stomach never breeds fine thoughts.'***
>
> ST JEROME

But don't eliminate all fat from your diet. Firstly, studies show you'll lose more weight if you include small amounts of fat in your diet. Plus your body needs one to two daily servings of essential fatty acids and monounsaturated fats each day for energy, eye function, brain-power, and for healthy skin and hair. Fats are also needed to absorb fat-soluble vitamins A, D, E and K which are important for vision, strong bones, and to help fight disease.

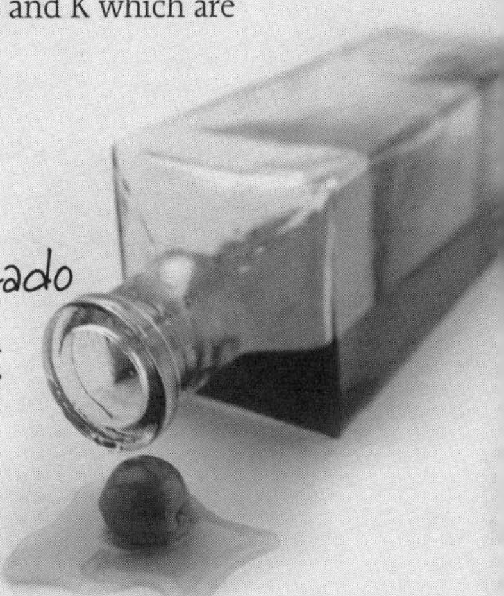

Here's where to get your daily fat:

80 g (quarter to one-half) of an avocado

One tablespoon of olive or rapeseed oils

10 g (half an ounce) butter

2 tablespoons of low fat mayo

2 tablespoons sunflower or pumpkin seeds

4–6 walnuts

3–4 tablespoons hummous

150 g oily fish such as sardines or mackerel

# How did it go?

**Q: I love my dressings and mayonnaise. Any good alternatives?**

A: Swap mayo for creamy roasted garlic and you could save yourself 80 calories and
8 g fat. Roasted garlic cloves make a rich, buttery substitute for dressing or
mayonnaise in potato, pasta and chicken salads (and no, they don't smell). Or try
spreading the paste on bread instead of butter. Take a head of garlic, trimmed to
expose the bulb and bake it sealed in foil with one tablespoon of water for 45
minutes at 200°C.

**Q: Cutting back on fat means cutting out the choccy doesn't it?
No can do!**

A: It doesn't mean banning it completely. Buy selection-pack minis and just treat
yourself to one a day. Or retrain your taste-buds by going for lower fat snack
alternatives such as half a banana sandwich, or fat-free popcorn. If you have a sweet
tooth, Turkish delight or jelly babies are virtually fat free!

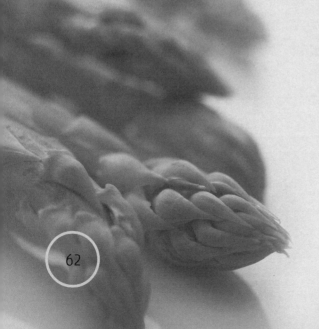

Defining idea...
**'No diet will remove all the
fat from your body because
the brain is entirely fat.
Without a brain, you might
look good, but all you could
do is run for public office.'**
GEORGE BERNARD SHAW

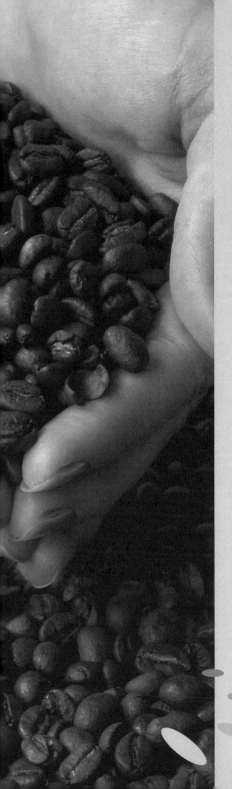

# 12

# Beans means lines

**Caffeine can dehydrate and age the skin, which can make cellulite worse. If you're a coffee fiend, it's time to switch to decaf.**

This will hurt if you're one of those people who can't face life without an espresso or five. But that black stuff is no friend to your behind.

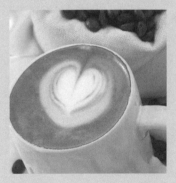

OK, most of us tend to find that a little caffeine fix makes us feel more alert, better able to concentrate and less tired. But too much caffeine can lead to anxiousness, restlessness, leave you feeling jittery and unable to sleep – and give you headaches, nausea or palpitations.

So what does caffeine have to do with cellulite, and more importantly why will your behind might thank you for cutting back on the cappuccino?

*Here's an idea for you...*
**Ditch that coffee and instead try starting your day with a large glass of freshly squeezed orange juice and a bowl of berries. This will boost your intake of vitamin C, which is important for the production of collagen and can strengthen the capillaries, which feed the skin. And better skin means smoother thighs.**

Firstly, caffeine can contribute to weight gain. (And there we were, thinking our little black cup was helping get us into our little black dress! *Au contraire*.) Apparently drinking two cups of coffee is enough to raise the levels of the stress hormone cortisol and insulin in your body, which is thought to accelerate ageing and encourage the body to store fat. Studies have shown that when coffee drinkers reduce their coffee intake, they lose weight, although it's not yet understood why this happens.

Plus when our blood sugar levels are raised and our insulin levels are disrupted, we're more likely to be tempted by sugary treats – that espresso may lead to a choccy croissant or two.

Caffeine is also bad for your skin because it impedes your blood circulation. Skin requires a regular blood supply to stay looking young and healthy. A lack of oxygen can lead to dark circles, puffiness, fine lines, poor colour. You know how your face looks after too many espressos and a few late nights...well, the skin on your behind is also being robbed of vital nutrients too, which means it's going to look dry and dehydrated – and that will make your cellulite worse.

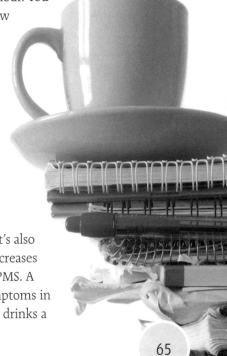

Caffeine also contributes to water retention; as it's a diuretic, it can dehydrate your body. When you're dehydrated, cells hold on to water – and your fat cells hold on to fluids, which, on your bottom and thighs, make your skin bulge out and look puffier and more dimply.

And if that hasn't put you off the black stuff, bear in mind it's also no friend if you're a PMS sufferer. That's because caffeine increases sleeplessness, anxiety and tension, which are symptoms of PMS. A study of over 200 college-age women found severe PMS symptoms in 60% of those who drank more than four cups of caffeinated drinks a

> *Try another idea...*
> **Cigarettes are bursting with nasty toxins that prematurely age your skin, as if you didn't know. So if you require tips on how to give up the evil weed, turn to IDEA 37, *Smoke gets in your eyes (and bottom and thighs)*.**

65

day. Coffee also causes your body to get rid of important nutrients, especially B vitamins, which are needed for energy, good skin and hair, healthy growth, and mood.

Defining idea...

**'Behind every successful woman is a substantial amount of coffee.'**
STEPHANIE PIRO, artist

It gets worse. Caffeine also destroys calcium – one cup of coffee removes about 6 mg of calcium from your body's stores. Experts have found that calcium is important in weight loss because it's thought to help prevent fat storage and boost metabolism. (You can increase the calcium in your diet with skimmed milk, cheddar cheese, fish, sesame seeds and dried figs. Other good sources include steamed tofu and nuts.)

### So how much is too much? How much caffeine are *you* drinking?

About 300 mg caffeine a day is 'a moderate' intake. One 190 ml cup of instant coffee contains about 100 mg, tea has 30–60 mg per cup and cola around 50 mg per can. So three mugs of tea per day plus one cup of coffee would give you almost your daily 'allowance'.

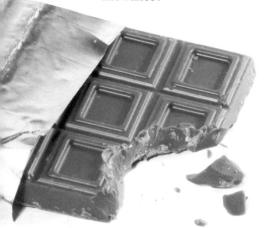

Best advice, then, is to cut down as much as you can – don't drink more than one or two cups a day – and look instead for healthy alternatives.

Bear in mind that chocolate also contains caffeine; in fact there's about 10 mg of caffeine in 50 g of milk chocolate – dark chocolate contains 28 mg per 50 g. There's more caffeine in a 125 g (4 oz) bar of dark chocolate that in a cup of instant coffee...so if you're serious about getting rid of cellulite, go easy on the chocolate.

# How did it go?

**Q: OK, you've convinced me. So are there any good alternatives to coffee?**

A: Try dandelion tea. Dandelion is rich in potassium and has long been used as a purifying tonic. You can buy ready-made teabags, or, alternatively, brew your own: pour boiling water over two teaspoons of dried dandelion leaves (or four teaspoons of freshly chopped ones) and steep for ten minutes. Strain, and drink. Or try green tea. It's made from the unfermented leaves of the tea plant, and has half the caffeine of coffee. It's rich in antioxidants, which can help mop up the free radicals that are associated with ageing. If you can only replace one cup of coffee with a cup of green tea you'll be doing your body a favour. Redbush tea is another good alternative. It contains on average less than half the tannin of regular tea. Research shows it's rich in disease-fighting antioxidants quercetin and luteolin. Plus it helps your body absorb vitamin C better. And it's delicious.

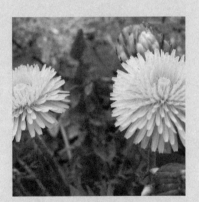

**Q: Help, I just can't give up my morning cup of coffee. How can I wake myself up without it?**

A: If you can't switch to decaf, or really can't function rationally without a morning brew, try to increase your intake of fluids. So for every caffeine-containing drink (such as tea, coffee or cola), make sure you have at least half a cup of water to counteract the diuretic effect.

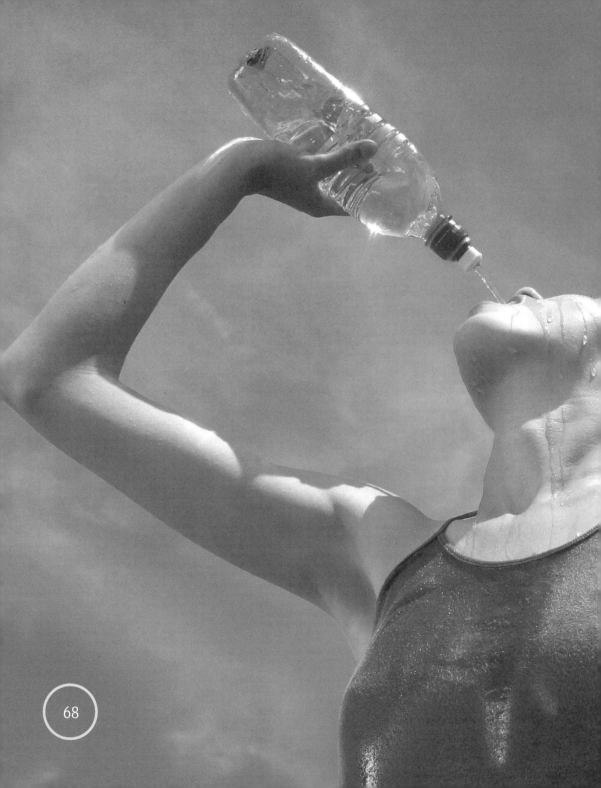

# 13

# Still waters

**Water is great for skin, and a few glasses a day may help reduce orange-peel thighs. Plus it's free. Get some water therapy today!**

If you need to ask why water could possibly reduce the appearance of cellulite, first look at a grape, then look at a raisin. Then look at your bottom. Capisce?

Water is involved in nearly every bodily function, from our circulation to our body temperature, and keeps our digestion and waste excretion working properly.

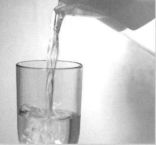

We need it to metabolise fat and flush waste from our cells. If our body is constantly dehydrated, it ages more quickly.

And being hydrated can help keep us slim; even being mildly dehydrated reduces our metabolic rate by 3% – that's about one pound of fat every six months!

So drinking plenty of water can help beat cellulite on several fronts.

It can be a great weight-loss tool. Many of us often confuse hunger with thirst, so we end up eating instead of drinking, increasing our calorie intake unnecessarily. Research shows that 75% of all hunger pangs are actually thirst, so if you get the munchies, try a glass of water instead – and save yourself calories. What's more, one study showed that you could increase your metabolic rate by about 30% by having a large glass of cold water after your meals. It comes down to a process called thermogenesis – that's the rate at which your body burns calories for digestion. Another study found that drinking two litres of water a day could help your body burn off an extra 150 calories a day.

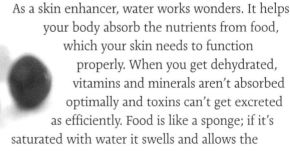

Here's an idea
for you...
**Book in regular 'water breaks'. Keep a big bottle or jug of water on your desk at work, set your computer to ping or send a reminder every twenty minutes or so, and make sure you have a glass or at least a big gulp. When your smoker colleagues head outside for a cigarette, that's your cue for an H$_2$O fix.**

As a skin enhancer, water works wonders. It helps your body absorb the nutrients from food, which your skin needs to function properly. When you get dehydrated, vitamins and minerals aren't absorbed optimally and toxins can't get excreted as efficiently. Food is like a sponge; if it's saturated with water it swells and allows the

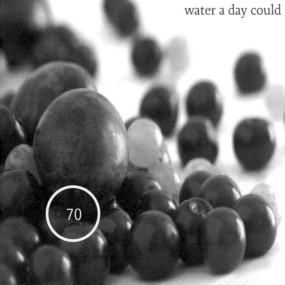

vitamins and minerals into your body – which can help heal you, boost your immune system and nourish your skin.

When you're dehydrated, your body effectively steals water from your skin to deliver to the more important organs, so skin is the first thing to suffer if you're not drinking enough.

Try another idea...
**Losing weight doesn't have to be painful and tedious. You'll barely notice the pounds drop with our tips in *IDEA 2, Want to know a secret?***

Drinking plenty of water can also help beat the water retention that contributes to cellulite. When you're dehydrated, or eat too much salt, for example, your body's cells hold on to the water it already has, fearing it won't get much more. The result is water swelling in your fat cells, which contributes to that dimply bottom look.

## How much should I drink?

Research shows that women who are adequately hydrated consume about 2.7 litres of fluids a day,

Defining idea...
*'When the well is dry, we know the worth of water.'*
BENJAMIN FRANKLIN

but that would include the fluid intake from food (which apparently accounts for as much as a third of our daily intake). Even bread and cheese contribute, apparently.

The British Dietetic Association recommends that the average 60 kg adult woman drink 1.5–2 litres (6–8 250 ml glasses) of fluids a day – plenty of which should be water. Alternatively aim for about 30 ml of water per kilo of body weight – or 1 litre for every 1,000 calories of food you consume.

The colour of your urine, though, is the best gauge – you're after a pale watery colour with a tinge of lemon. Yellow urine means you need to drink more.

Make sure you're well hydrated at all times. Carry a bottle around with you and sip regularly. Match every caffeine beverage or alcoholic drink with a glass of water. When you're exercising drink about two glasses (400–600 ml) two to three hours before you start your work-out. Going out to eat? Take a tip from the Americans, and ask for a jug of iced tap water on your table. Get into the habit of drinking a glass of water as soon as you wake up, too. And always knock back a large glass of the stuff at bedtime if you've been out drinking. It can take the edge off a hangover headache.

Another good way to beat fluid retention is to cut back on salt, and up your potassium intake (it helps counteract the effect of sodium). Fresh fruit, veg, and wholegrains will help rebalance the salts in your body, and help eliminate excess fluid in your fat pockets.

## How did it go?

**Q: I know it's good for me, but I find water so boring. Do I really have to drink eight glasses of the stuff a day?**
A: The good news is that US experts now say you don't have to get your eight glasses of fluids a day from water alone. Milk, tea, squashes and juices, even coffee count too. However, avoid fizzy drinks or you'll be loading your body with sugar, and possibly additives. Milk is great, as it provides calcium, but be aware you're adding calories too. Aim for the purest drinks – freshly squeezed orange juice, smoothies, herbal teas, and tart up your water with a squeeze of lemon or lime.

**Q: Warm water? Cold water? Does it matter?**
A: Drink it cool if you can. Drinking water from the fridge or served with ice can boost your energy levels as well as help you lose weight. Apparently your body can't absorb cold fluids very easily, so it has to increase energy production with every sip you take just to warm the fluid up.

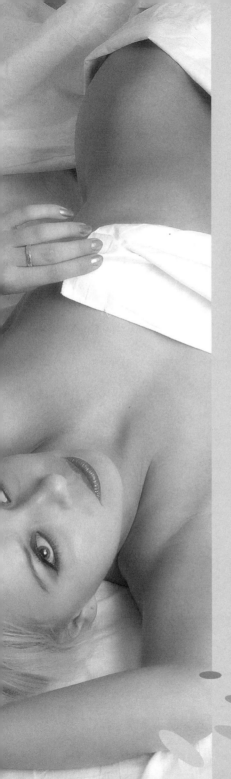

# 14

# Top gear

**As you age, your metabolism slows down, which means more body fat, and a saggier bottom and thighs as the years go by. Try some strategies to rev up your body chemistry.**

Were you at the back of the queue when they were handing out metabolic rates? 'It's not me, it's my metabolism' is an oft-given excuse for erring on the lardy side.

To a certain extent, your metabolic rate is genetic. Experts say that the rate at which a person burns up calories can vary as much as 25% – that's between people of the same weight.

Your age also affects the rate at which you burn calories. Between the ages of 30 and 80, muscle mass decreases by 40–50%, which reduces your strength and slows down your metabolism.

So, if you've drawn the short straw, and you're gaining weight – and cellulite – as a result, it's time to get tough on your metabolism.

Here's an idea for you...

Drinking 2 litres of still water a day can help your body burn off an extra 150 calories according to one study. It's thought to stimulate the sympathetic nervous system and increase the metabolic rate.

Start by working out how many calories you actually need, based on your metabolic rate. Remember, you gain weight when you take in more calories than you expend.

First, calculate your basal metabolic rate (BMR) – this is the rate at which your body burns energy even when you're not doing anything.

Your BMR = weight in kilos × 2 × 11 (if you prefer to work in pounds that will be your weight in pounds × 11)

So, if you're 65 kilos, your BMR = 65 × 2 × 11 = 1,430

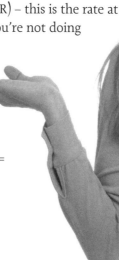

**Now work out how many extra calories you expend according to your lifestyle:**

■ Inactive or sedentary: BMR × 20%.

■ Fairly active, i.e. you walk and take exercise once or twice a week: BMR × 30%.

■ Moderately active, i.e. you exercise two or three times a week: BMR × 40%.

■ Active (you exercise hard more than three times a week): BMR × 50%.

■ Very active (you exercise hard every day): BMR × 70%.

*Try another idea...*

**Are you addicted to crisps and salty snacks? Do you live on convenience foods? Additives, sugar and salt can make cellulite worse. Clean up your cupboards with IDEA 16, *There's a rat in the kitchen.***

So if you're a fairly active 65 kg woman, your additional calorie requirement is 1,430 × 30% = 429.

Add this to your BMR to find out how many calories you need a day: 1,430 + 429 = 1,859. So if you eat more than 1,900 calories and don't increase your activity levels, you'll gain weight.

# What's the best way to boost your metabolic rate?

Defining idea...

*'Genius depends on dry air, on clear skies – that is, on rapid metabolism, on the possibility of drawing again and again on great, even tremendous quantities of strength.'*
FRIEDRICH NIETZSCHE

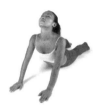

### Exercise

Move more: incorporate regular aerobic and weight-bearing exercise into your week (running, hill walking or weight training will do). When you increase the amount of lean tissue in your body, you use up more calories even when you're just sitting there; muscle uses more calories than fat does. Aim for 30–40 minute sessions, four or five times a week.

### Eat regularly, and don't fast

When you eat less, your metabolism drops because your body tries to conserve energy in case its food supply is about to run out. Small, regular meals are better than scoffing a big meal then eating nothing for hours.

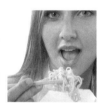

### Eat protein

Eating protein uses more calories than other foodstuffs. If you're doing an aerobic workout three to five times a week you need more protein – about 1.1 g of protein for every kilo of body weight. If you're sedentary you need about 0.8 g per kilo of body weight. (As a guide, you get about 44 g of protein in an average lean steak, and about 25 g in a portion of lean chicken.)

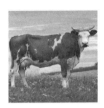

### Have a steak occasionally

Red meat and dairy produce contain conjugated linoleic acid (CLA). Research has shown this may increase the amount of lean tissue in your body, which boosts metabolic rate.

### Go exotic

Add some chillies to your dishes – apparently they can raise your metabolic rate by about 50% for up to two or three hours after a meal.

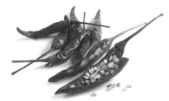

### Have a pre- and post-exercise nibble

One recent study found that people who performed gentle resistance exercise within two hours of eating a light, carb-based meal boosted their metabolic rate, and burned the food off quicker than those who didn't exercise afterwards. Plus, if you aim to eat something within half an hour of finishing a workout you'll increase your metabolic rate further. After exercising, your body will be low in energy. Replace it quickly and you'll keep your metabolism higher.

### Have a coffee break

Caffeine can boost your metabolic rate – partly because it increases your heart rate and also because it makes you fidgety! Don't drink more than two or three cups a day though. Alternatively, try green tea. Studies show that drinking a cup of the green stuff twice daily could help you burn about 70 calories more each day – that's about 3.5 kg in a year! Researchers believe it's the catechins (antioxidants) and other flavonoids in green tea that help boost your metabolism.

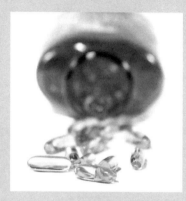

## How did it go?

**Q: Do any supplements help with weight loss?**

A: Possibly. US research found that vitamin B12 may help eliminate extra pounds; in studies, people who increased their B12 intake were more likely to lose weight than those who didn't. This vitamin may help you burn calories more effectively. Alternatively up your intake of vitamin B12 through diet: six oysters provides 16 mcg, while a trout fillet or salmon steak will net you about 5 mcg.

**Q: Could cold temperatures in winter affect my metabolism?**

A: In theory, yes, your metabolism does pick up a bit in the winter, because your body expends more energy trying to keep warm. Plus it rises if you move around more in an attempt to keep your body warm. Don't let rain and sleet keep you from the gym though. Exercise not only boosts your metabolism, it also lifts a low mood – which may help fight the winter blues and comfort eating.

> Defining idea...
> **'Energy and persistence conquer all things.'**
> BENJAMIN FRANKLIN

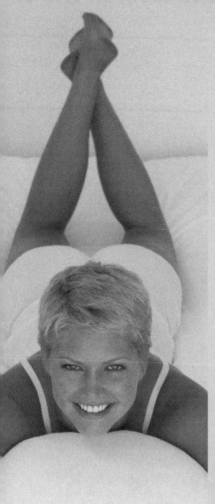

## 15

# Brown girl in the ring

**Cellulite looks less obvious on bronzed legs. If you can't beat it...hide it with a fake tan!**

There's no denying it, a golden body is a great confidence booster. You just tend to look longer, leaner, more toned with a bit of colour.

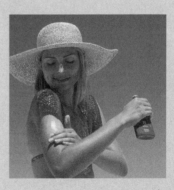

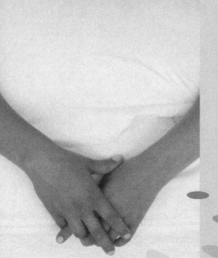

Faking it is so much safer than baking in the sun. And many of us would agree that we would be less tempted to soak up the rays if we arrived on holiday with a bit of colour.

It's also brilliant at helping disguise cellulite – fake tan somehow seems to even out those lumps and bumps. Plus the prep work you do before you apply it – exfoliating, moisturising and so on – helps hydrate the area, remove dead skin cells and even out skin-texture. So cellulitey skin can look better already.

Applying fake tan used to be a messy, smelly old business. And the shades were questionable.

Mercifully, gone are the days of George Hamilton-style tans in a shade of tangerine that smelt of something you'd keep under the sink.

*Here's an idea for you...*

**Fake tanning doesn't have to be a messy, painstaking business. You can buy packets of nifty little self-tan wipes, which you just rub over your skin, and a golden tan appears in a few hours. Keep a packet in your handbag, just in case you need to undress and impress pronto.**

These days fake tans are sophisticated, easy to use, quick-drying and incredibly effective. They're a great way to prepare your body for your two weeks in the sun, or cover up pasty white bits when you're wearing that sundress/mini-skirt/strappy number.

Try another idea...
**Here's a zero-effort approach to cellulite busting – the cellulite-busting patch you stick on and leave! Find out how (on earth) it works in IDEA 52, *Getting plastered*.**

The magic ingredient is DHA (dihydroxyacetene), which turns the skin brown by oxidizing amino acids in the skin. And manufacturers usually add lots of other lovely softening, toning, hydrating ingredients too.

Fake tans come in mousses, creams, gels and lotions. You can either apply them yourself – home tans tend to last up to four or five days. Or you can go the professional route and visit a specialist, who might put you in a booth and spray you with the stuff. Salon tans tend to last longer – some claim theirs last between a week and a fortnight.

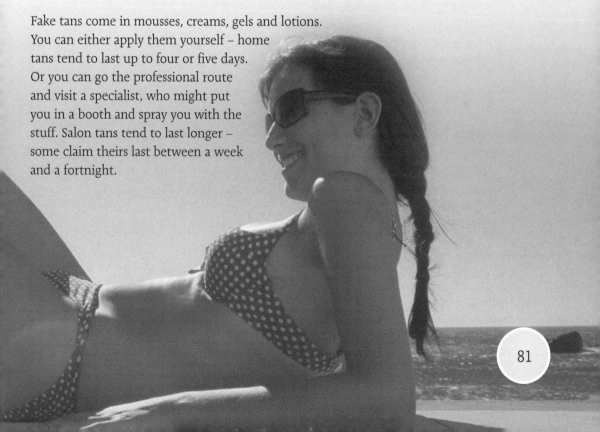

81

**A salon is the best route if you want an all-over tan without the hassle of doing it yourself. Best salon choices include St Tropez, Guinot and Clarins.**

Defining idea...

*'I will not retire while I've still got my legs and my make-up box.'*
BETTE DAVIS

Here's what to expect if you're a salon tan virgin. You disrobe (and usually pop on a pair of charming paper pants), after which the therapist exfoliates you, and slaps on handfuls of goo, covering you thoroughly. She'll then leave you there for up to an hour while the tanner works its magic, and she then removes the excess. When you shower the next day (if you can leave it that long) you look fantastic. Make sure you wear dark clothes to avoid staining on your clothes.

Many fake tans take a few days to look beautifully natural, so if you're preparing for a special do, book your treatment a few days prior to the event.

*And always remember that a fake tan won't protect you from the sun so you still need sunscreen.*

If you're using a self-tanner at home, make sure you patch test the area beforehand to avoid an allergic reaction. Don't be tempted to go too dark; always choose one that matches your natural skin tone. The best tried-and-tested self-tanners include those by Decleor, Ambre Solaire, St-Tropez and Lancaster.

**Follow the three golden rules: *exfoliate*, *moisturise* and *layer*.**

- Start by exfoliating the area with a body scrub, loofah or flannel. Apply exfoliator with circular movements (it helps boost circulation). Make sure you pay particular attention to heels, knees and elbows where the skin is rougher. A cheaper option is Epsom salts – which will help to deep-cleanse your skin. Just fill a cup with salts and add enough water to make a paste. Massage over your skin, then rinse off.

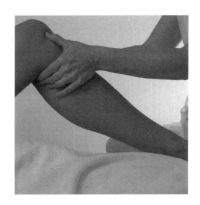

- Always moisturise after exfoliating. Leave the moisturiser on for about fifteen minutes before you apply your fake tan so it doesn't interfere with the active ingredient in fake tanning products.

- Remove excess moisturiser with a damp flannel before you apply the tanning product – especially on bony areas such as knees, elbows and ankles – it'll prevent any uneven tanning.

- Apply the fake tan, smothering it on as you would a moisturiser. Don't forget backs of knees and hands, and your inner thighs.

Defining idea...

*'The average man is more interested in a woman who is interested in him than he is in a woman with beautiful legs.'*
MARLENE DIETRICH

- Then build up gradually. You don't need as much where your skin is thinner as the colour will stay longer here.

- Tan usually appears about three or four hours later – if you find you have streaks, try exfoliating the area.

- Avoid swimming or having a shower for about twelve hours after a treatment.

- Moisturise your body well over the next few days; it'll help prolong your fake tan.

# How did it go?

**Q: Argh! I've just finished my fake tan and have orange palms! What can I do to salvage my skin colour?**

A: Oh no! Nightmare. Your options include wearing gloves, or standing clench-fisted for the next few weeks – or alternatively try rubbing the juice of a lemon over your palms; it's a natural bleach so should do the trick. Another great tip is to shampoo your hair as the detergents in the products help fade the colour.

**Q: I was sensible – applied fake tan before I went in the sun, smothered on sunscreen, but obviously missed a few bits, which are now lobster red. What should I do now?**

A: If these red bits are stinging, add a couple of spoonfuls of baking soda to your bath to help relieve the pain. If you burned on, say, your nose, or by the edge of your bikini strap, use one of those high protection sticks (which are about factor 30): this will cut out about 96% of the sun's burning rays, and reduce the discomfort. Using an after-sun product once you're out of the sun will also prolong a tan and replace lost moisture in the skin. Look for added vitamin E – it helps protect against premature skin ageing.

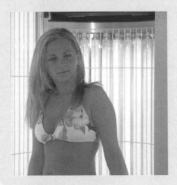

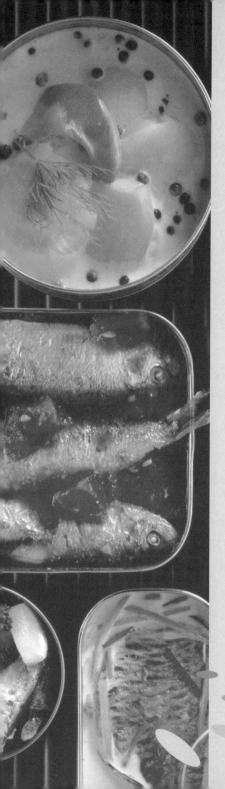

# 16

# There's a rat in the kitchen

**Are you sure you know what you're putting in your mouth? Additives, salt and sugar all conspire to make your bottom crinkly. Start saying no to processed foods.**

Convenience foods are so darn handy, but are often laden with fat and calories — or worse.

You know that eating surplus calories makes wobbly thighs flabbier. Start upgrading the overall quality of the food you eat, and you can improve skin and help smooth orange-peel thighs.

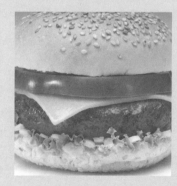

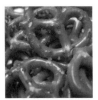

## Salt

Salt is no friend to a cellulite-ridden girl because it encourages your body to hold on to water, which can cause bloating. When your cells hold on to water it causes that dimpling under the skin that we know as cellulite. Your body also needs plenty of water to help keep your kidneys working – diluting your body's waste products and helping eliminate them.

Here's an idea for you...

**If you want to minimise the cellulite while posing for holiday snaps, hold yourself in a way that disguises excess curves. Stand up and pivot slightly on your feet so your body, including your shoulders, is at a slight angle. Put your hands on your hips to make your waist look smaller. Overall it'll take inches off your body.**

**Time for some salt busters:**

- Watch your salt intake; have no more than 6 g (or 2.4 g sodium) of salt a day.

- Cut back on processed foods – beware stock, sauces and soups as the processed versions are salt-laden. Instead cook from scratch. That way you're in control of your salt intake.

- Aim to drink plenty of fluids every day (at least eight glasses) and potassium-rich fruit and veg, to help dilute the salt.

- Use fresh herbs, spices, lemon or mustard instead of salt to flavour your food.

- As a rule, foods that contain more than 0.5 g of sodium per 100 g serving (or 1.25 g of salt or more per 100 g) are considered high in salt. Foods than contain less than 0.1 g sodium (0.25 g salt) per 100 g are considered low-sodium foods.

■ Be a savvy shopper. Some products only label sodium content, not salt content. To work out your salt intake multiply the sodium figure by 2.5 to find the amount of salt. So if there's 0.6 g sodium in 100 g and you're eating 300 g of it, you're getting 4.5 g salt (0.6 × 3 = 1.8 g sodium; 1.8 g sodium × 2.5 = 4.5 g salt).

> *Try another idea...*
> **Tempted by a quick-fix crash diet? Step away from that crispbread. Very low-calorie programmes may make cellulite worse. Find a better alternative in IDEA 24, *The big easy*.**

 ## Sugar

Sugar is high in calories, plus, when we eat sugary foods, it can cause blood sugar levels to surge, which triggers the release of insulin, which encourages fat storage.

Skin experts also say that eating a high-sugar diet is bad for your skin; it has been linked to premature ageing. Sugar may have an inflammatory effect on our tissues and can cause the collagen to become hard and less elastic. And if the collagen in your skin gets becomes, this can contribute to the puckering effect on your bottom and thighs.

**Try some sugar busters:**

■ Cut back on sugary foods – rather than banning sweet treats, limit them to a once weekly indulgence.

■ Watch the labels for hidden sugars – the baddies include glucose syrup and dextrose.

■ Start label watching – aim for less than 2 g sugar per 100 g of a foodstuff.

■ Watch your soft drinks – they're often full of sugar. Stick to natural juices or smoothies instead.

- Sweeten foods with fresh/stewed fruit or dried fruit – they're also more nutritious.

- Try to have no more than 10% of your total daily calories from sugar (that's a maximum of 20 g a day if you're eating about 2,000 calories daily).

Defining idea...

**'Life expectancy would grow by leaps and bounds if green vegetables smelled as good as bacon.'**
DOUG LARSON, Olympic gold medallist

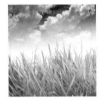 Pesticides

Some scientists claim that the pesticide residues and additives found in many conventional foods actually interfere with our metabolism, disrupt our hormone balance (which is necessary to regulate our weight), and increase our appetite, all of which can make us gain pounds.

They argue that by switching to a purer, organic diet, you can help restore your body's metabolism and lose weight more quickly.

**Pesticide busters:**

- Choose organic where possible.

- Keep your fat intake down (apparently you take in more chemical calories from fats compared to carbs).

- Eat plenty of soluble fibre (beans, lentils, pulses, oats, apples, oranges) to soak up chemical calories from other ingredients.

- Cut back on savoury snacks, desserts, sweets and snack bars – they're often full of colours, preservatives or additives.

- Cut off all visible fat as you prepare fish or meat. Chemical calories are thought to accumulate in animal fat.

- Cook vegetables where possible – even light cooking helps wash off many chemicals.

# How did it go?

**Q: I can't afford to go completely organic. What should I splash out on?**

A: Most experts say fatty foods, such as meat, dairy and oily fish, should be organic (or 'wild' fish). Spinach, lettuce, cabbage and potatoes, and perishable soft fruits such as strawberries are more likely to be treated with chemicals than other fruit and veg. Peel fruits – you lose some of the nutrients in the skin, but a peeled apple generally contains fewer pesticides.

**Q: What kinds of foods contain 'hidden' sugars?**

A: A can of cola has about seven teaspoons of sugar, a small can of baked beans has about two teaspoons. One tablespoon of tomato ketchup has about one teaspoon of sugar. And a small bowl of frosted cereal contains about three teaspoons. Even a fruit yoghurt which you'd be forgiven for thinking is 'healthy' has about three teaspoons of sugar. Start reading labels.

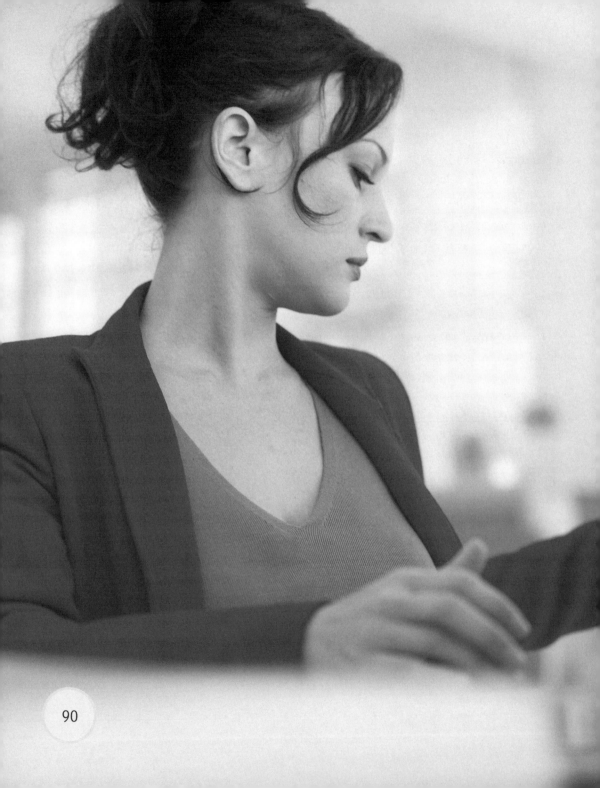

## 17

# Be a mistress of disguise

**Some clothes actually draw attention to cellulite. Learn what to wear to make the most of your assets.**

If you reckon figure-hugging jeans, white Lycra and a snug waistband are helping accentuate your curves and distract from your cellulite, think again. You could be making matters worse.

What are you wearing today? And what is it doing for your cellulite? Is it cleverly disguising it or making you look like you have spoonfuls of cottage cheese in your pockets?

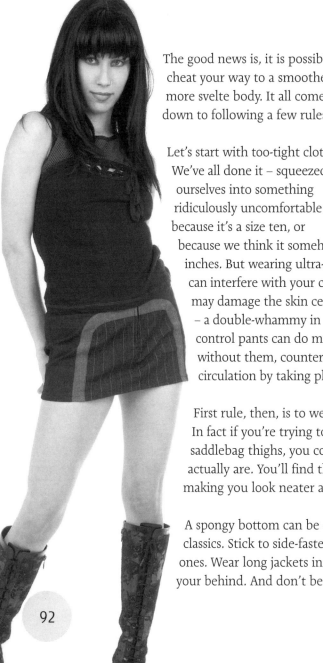

The good news is, it is possible to cheat your way to a smoother, more svelte body. It all comes down to following a few rules.

Let's start with too-tight clothes. We've all done it – squeezed ourselves into something ridiculously uncomfortable because it's a size ten, or because we think it somehow eradicates a few of the gruesome inches. But wearing ultra-tight clothes and even control undies can interfere with your circulation and lymph drainage, and this may damage the skin cells, and also exacerbate water retention – a double-whammy in your war on cellulite. (Having said that, control pants can do miraculous things, so if you can't live without them, counteract their potential ill-effects on your circulation by taking plenty of exercise!)

First rule, then, is to wear the right size clothes for your body. In fact if you're trying to hide a generous bottom and saddlebag thighs, you could even wear a size bigger than you actually are. You'll find that trousers hang more flatteringly, making you look neater and trimmer.

A spongy bottom can be camouflaged with a few wardrobe classics. Stick to side-fastening trousers instead of front-fastening ones. Wear long jackets instead of cropped ones; they'll cover your behind. And don't be tempted by drainpipe trousers

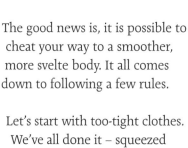

*Here's an idea for you...*

**Draw the eye away from your rear end with bright Pucci-style numbers – gorgeous billowy tops in bold colours can take unwanted attention away from your thighs.**

however great they look on Kate Moss; stick to wide legs that make your tush altogether more petite. Hipsters are a big-bottomed girl's best friend – they can virtually cut it in half visually – and can be really flattering whatever your age as they create the illusion of having smaller hips. But avoid an expanse of flesh 'overhang' as this can ruin the effect. Team hipsters with a floaty top. And experiment with a boot-leg cut – it's even more flattering as it makes your legs look longer and slimmer.

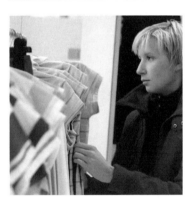

Try another idea...

**Exercise has proven effects on cellulite. Try our softly-softly approach to firmer thighs in IDEA 5, *Keep on running.***

Tailored clothes tend to look better on generously proportioned behinds so splash out on some quality classics – you'll notice the difference instantly. Legs and hips beleaguered by cellulite can be enhanced by tailored flares and floaty palazzo pants or A-line skirts; these are also great for disguising saddlebags.

Hands up anyone with cellulitey arms? Isn't it awful how those batwings jiggle like blancmange? Best advice, then, is to throw out any tops or blouses that show an expanse of wobbly flesh – tight vest tops or halternecks, puffy or capped sleeves: bin them all. Instead stick to lovely floaty sleeves with fluted cuffs. And buy T-shirts or jersey tops with three-quarter length sleeves instead.

If your cellulite tends to lurk around a flabby waist and tummy, you'd do well to invest in a thick belt. Wear it low slung over a fitted top and it automatically draws the eye inwards and makes your middle look neater. Don't wear it too tight, though, or you'll bulge out the sides! Stick to low deep V-necks or wrap-around tops, dresses or cardigans to cinch in that waist. Ruched tops can make your torso look slimmer.

## Other rules for cellulite-sufferers

- Stick to small patterns rather than unflattering big ones.

- Avoid panty lines at all costs.

- Never wear tight leggings.

- For waists try deep V-necks and corset tops.

- Avoid spray-on Lycra – boy, can it show up the bulges.

- Stick to floaty fabrics such as chiffon or tailored lines in natural fibres such as linen or cotton.

- Seek out textured fabrics. They can help to 'break up' flesh. Think linen, wool or even crinkled man-made fabrics.

Investing in some fabulous and clever lingerie can help fast-track you to Monroesque curves. You can take inches off your waist, flatten your middle and add a cup size to your bust with a few strategic undies.

Defining idea...

'**If God wanted us to be naked, why did he invent sexy lingerie?'**
SHANNEN DOHERTY, actress

Splash out on a fabulous corset that nips in your waist and lifts your bust. Slip into a pair of front-flattering pants. Reinforced thongs are a godsend: these flatten your tummy without the cursed VPL.

## How did it go?

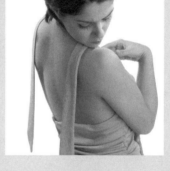

**Q: Will I look slimmer and more toned in black?**

A: Depends. Not if it's too-tight Lycra or an unflattering cut that makes you look bulky. General slimming rules say the longer the streak you create, the better. Dark colours certainly can minimise the bulges, and you can refine your silhouette by sticking to one colour – and pretty much any colour. In summer you can still dress to create the illusion of being longer and leaner if you're dressed head to foot in the same shade, even white.

**Q: What about when it's hot and I want to wear shorts and crop tops?**

A: Where possible, choose lined clothes or natural fabrics that don't hug you unforgivingly. Linen trousers or shorts are ideal, particularly in summer – they drop flatteringly, however hot and sweaty you are beneath. Wide-leg shorts that skim the knee are more becoming than tight ultra-brief shorts. Avoid any too-tight teeny T-shirts that cause dimply flesh to bulge out.

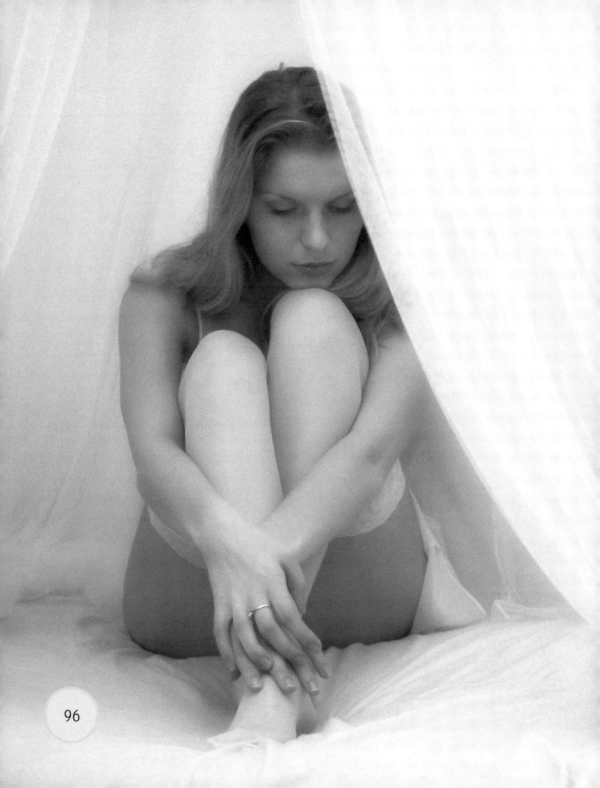

# 18

# Come to bed thighs

**Soft lighting in the bedroom can make all the difference to your confidence. In the dark no one can see your cellulite, so light some candles and snuggle up.**

Nothing cools a woman's ardour more than the thought of a man coming face to face with her cellulitey body. (Though we'd argue that once he's close enough actually to see your cellulite, it's going to be the last thing on his mind.)

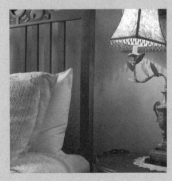

Still, most of us would feel more confident if we had a few tricks up our sleeve to upstage our cellulite. Here are a few:

## Make the bedroom work

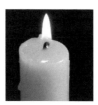

Create a seductive boudoir and you'll guarantee he won't be fixated by cellulitey thighs. That means thinking of sounds, smells, textures and first impressions.

**Here's an idea for you...**

Hot day? Hot date? If you want to reveal some flesh without displaying your cellulitey arms or legs, show off your back instead. Try a backless dress or long-sleeved top with a plunging back. Keep your back looking toned (with Pilates, backstroke and yoga) and smooth. Keep it smooth by exfoliating regularly with a long-handled loofah, and by soaking in moisturising bath oils.

■ Swap your bright 100 watt bulb for a more atmospheric 40 or 60 watt one. Or try tea lights or scented candles.

■ 'Set' your bedroom. Display pictures of yourself looking gorgeous (happy/slim/firm) on the mantelpiece or by the bed; drape a slinky negligée over a hanger, stockings across the back of the chair, satin slippers – you know the kind of thing. Make sure the room is clear of clutter.

■ Fill your room with fresh flowers (freesias are deliciously intoxicating), or bowls of fruit (pomegranates symbolise fertility) or light aromatherapy candles.

■ Make the bed work with fantastic crisp, cotton sheets. Add layers and textures – think cashmere throws, fur blankets and plump cushions (which you can strategically place over yourself).

■ Have mellow music ready, something deep and soulful.

## Smell: Don't forget your perfume

- Why? Because our 'odour memory' is housed in the same part of the brain that controls emotional and sexual response...

- Choose your fragrance wisely; tuberose is relaxing and sensuous and is said to help increase happiness.

- Hyacinth has been found to increase sensuality.

- Fragrances such as jasmine, tuberose, ylang-ylang, patchouli, sandalwood, rose, cardamom, cedarwood, cinnamon and clary sage are known for their aphrodisiac qualities.

- Use your perfume to its best advantage. Spray eau de toilette across your body a few times, then add a touch of eau de parfum – either on your wrist or on the dip of your collar bone.

- Spritz it on to your lingerie (be careful with light colours as some perfumes stain). Or spray into the air and walk in a mist of fragrance.

## Confidence tips

- Look less lumpy instantly by improving your posture. Imagine there's string pulling you up from the centre of your head. Your stomach should be pressed flat. Relax your shoulders down into your back. Many of us round our shoulders, which makes breasts look droopy and our tummy protrude.

- Make a mental note of your most attractive qualities. Think about it long enough and you'll come up with dozens. Honestly. Believe them.

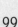

99

- Visualise yourself as a beautiful, sensuous woman; rehearse scary encounters/conversations in the mirror before the event.

- Pop a Bach's flower remedy on your tongue to boost self-esteem. Try larch, it's for those 'who secretly know they have the ability – but fear failure', or gentian, which helps 'dispel despondency'.

*Try another idea...*

**Splash out on some figure-flattering hosiery – some is made to combat cellulite and make legs look slimmer! Turn to IDEA 36, *The lady vanishes.***

## Quick beauty tricks

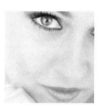

- If you've got time, try a twenty-minute workout before your date – a short run or walk uphill, anything that gets you out of breath and your legs moving. By boosting your circulation you'll improve skin tone and look more radiant.

- Set aside five or ten minutes to exfoliate your skin to remove surface dead skin cells, then moisturise – it'll help 'plump' up the skin.

- Make use of bronzer and moisturising creams with light-reflecting particles; they can make legs look more even-textured and glowing.

- Try a kitten heel rather than flatties to make your legs look longer and leaner.

- Don't underestimate the power of a pair of floaty bedroom palazzo pants (think Hollywood legends Grace Kelly and Katharine Hepburn).

*Defining idea...*

*'My wife was afraid of the dark...then she saw me naked and now she's afraid of the light.'*
RODNEY DANGERFIELD, comedian

## Night attire tricks

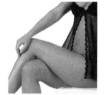

- Don't go too skimpy. Always buy knickers a size bigger so you're not spilling over the top.

- Ditto bra (unless you're aiming for that 'cup spilleth over' look).

- Satin is great as it skims over your bits. Pale pink suits most people's colouring.

- Distract from your dimply bottom by drawing his eyes to other bits – such as your neckline. Wear a beautiful necklace or choker.

- Make your neck look longer with long dangly earrings.

## How did it go?

**Q: How do I get his attention to shift from my thighs to my cleavage?**
A: Flaunt it. Nell Gwynne firmness isn't that difficult to achieve. But make sure you're wearing the right sized bra. Get fitted: you'll be amazed at what the right size can do for you. Dusting bronzer with light reflecting particles over your cleavage will make your breasts 'pop out' and give them a youthful curve.

**Q: Can you suggest any good exercises to emphasise my bust – and keep his eyes there?**
A: This posture-booster will make sure his eyes stay above the waist. Raise your shoulders to your ears, squeeze as hard as you can as if you're doing an exaggerated shrug, then drop them. Try to squeeze your shoulder blades together behind you, then relax them. It's a great way to keep your shoulders back and bust perky.

101

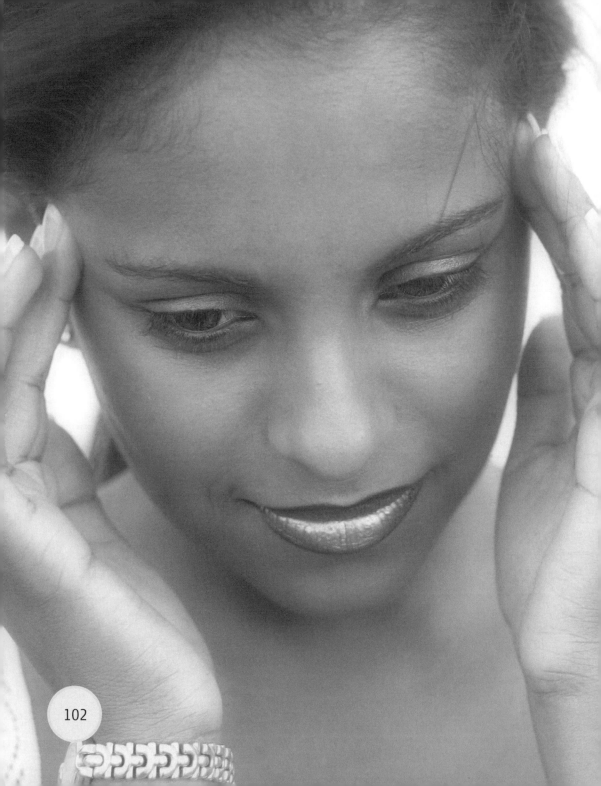

# 19

# The big chill

**The stress hormone cortisol can make cellulite worse. Time for some simple stress reduction strategies.**

We know what you're thinking. Stress and cellulite? Cellulite and stress? What on earth does stress have to do with cellulite? The answer is: more than you think.

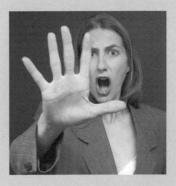

Let me ask you a question. Does your mood ever affect what you eat? Or do you ever use food to boost your mood? Most women out there are probably nodding frantically, 'Oooh, yes, absolutely.' And let's face it, who hasn't been known to grab an eclair/chocolate bar/ice-cream sundae in order to brighten up a bad or troublesome day?

The truth is stress can contribute to cellulite on two levels. Firstly, being in a state of stress may actually make you fat. This might seem strange to you: how can this be so, given that many people actually find it hard to eat when they're under short periods of stress, and often end up losing weight?

Sure, that happens. But *long-term* stress can make you fat because it often increases the appetite for carbohydrate-rich 'comfort' foods.

It's a hormone thing. Experts have found that the adrenal hormone cortisol, which is released when you are stressed, can increase fat storage in the abdominal area (where many of us get cellulite). That's because the deep fat in the abdomen contains receptors that the cortisol prefers.

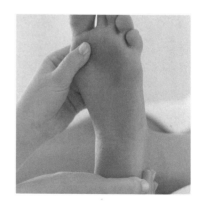

Cortisol basically boosts your appetite, making you want to eat vast quantities, and making you fancy sweets and carbohydrate-rich foods too. These cause insulin levels to spike and then plummet, which may leave you feeling hungrier than ever – and eating again.

And stress can also compromise your overall nutrition because it makes the food pass more quickly through your digestive system, which means less of it is actually absorbed.

*Try another idea...*

**How's your pain threshold? If the thought of having cellulite-busting injections in your buttocks doesn't make you flinch, turn to IDEA 30, *There's a hole in my buttocks, dear Henry, dear Henry.***

Secondly, stress also has an ageing effect on your skin. Stress causes hormonal changes in your body, which affect the function of cells in your vital organs. These changes are then reflected in your skin.

The key, then, is to seize control of your stress levels before they end up on your tummy, bum and thighs.

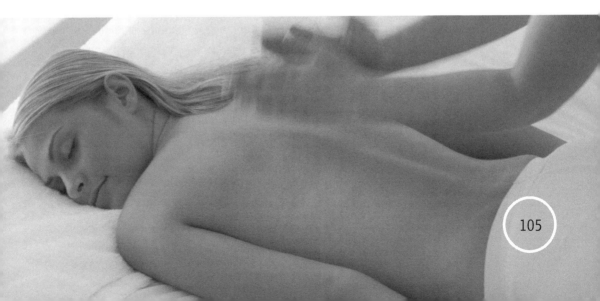

105

**Start by perfecting some relaxation techniques.**

■ Make sure you relax for 5 or 10 minutes before meals in order to prepare your digestive system; food will be absorbed and metabolised more efficiently if you're calmer. Go for a walk, sit and meditate for ten minutes, have a bath before supper.

■ Don't let chores get on top of you. Write achievable, realistic to-do lists for daily/weekly/monthly chores.

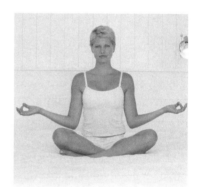

■ Keep your surroundings decluttered: every day have a 15-minute tidy up before bedtime – put your clothes out for the morning, make sure the supper dishes are cleaned up and put away. And regularly set aside 20 minutes to an hour for one task, such as tidying that drawer/shelf/cupboard/room.

■ Get some exercise: ideally try to manage 30 minutes of moderate exercise at least five days of the week – walking to work/shops/school, and gardening. Swimming, dancing, Pilates and yoga are relaxing and body-firming too. Studies show that regular exercise can reduce your risk of depression and anxiety and one study found that 30 minutes a day – broken up into 10-minute sessions – was enough to improve mood and regulate emotions.

■ Pamper yourself with a haircut, pedicure, manicure, massage, leg wax. Savour a night in – slap on a face pack, pour a glass of wine, curl up in front of a great video. Splurge on a spa day or weekend away.

■ Surround yourself with blues and greens. Blue is a calming, serene colour which has been found to lower blood pressure and pulse rate and help reduce stress. Green is great if you can't sleep, or feel over-anxious.

- Put uplifting photos in your 'stress zones'. Clip a picture of your latest holiday on the dashboard to calm you when you're stuck in traffic. Place pictures of happy times or places on your desk.

- Perfect a mantra: in times of stress or anxiety, take 5 minutes out for some meditation. Silently repeat a soothing word or phrase, such as 'peace', while taking slow, deep breaths through your nose.

- Have a laugh. Studies show that people who laugh have significantly lower levels of another stress hormone, epinephrine. Watch some funny videos or get your friends over regularly for a fun evening.

- Have a massage. Studies have shown that deep-pressure massage stimulates the nerves that cause our levels of the stress hormones cortisol and epinephrine to go down. And it causes the levels of two mood-regulating brain chemicals to rise.

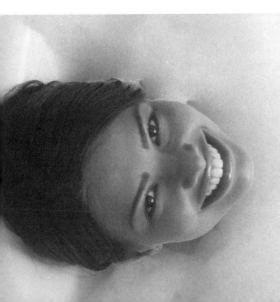

# How did it go?

### Q: How can I find the time to relax?

A: Try this 5-minute 'relaxation' exercise every day. Lie on the floor or the bed in a relaxed position, and breathe in deeply for a count of six. Hold for six, then breathe out for six. Repeat six times, letting go of tension throughout your body as you do so. Focus on each body part in turn, gradually releasing the stiffness: feel the anxiety leave your body. Then as you breathe in, bring your arms over your head to stretch out your body. As your breathe out, bring them back by your sides again. Repeat. Then lie still for a few moments, before you get up slowly.

### Q: What can I munch to counteract stress without eating my body weight in biscuits?

A: Eat vitamin C-rich foods (satsumas, kiwi fruit, broccoli) to counteract the harmful effect of stress hormones and boost immunity. Include foods rich in B vitamins in your diet – you need them for making anti-stress hormones. Try bananas, wholegrain bread, beans and nuts. Eating essential fatty acids found in nuts, seeds and oily fish, and vitamin B6-rich foods (such as bananas, chicken, sunflower seeds) can also help prevent mood disorders. Tryptophan-rich foods such as turkey and cottage cheese can help you sleep if stress is interfering with your sleep. If you must comfort-eat, stick to dark chocolate (70% cocoa), as it's rich in antioxidants, and contains various minerals. It contains phenylethylamine which releases the feel-good chemical dopamine.

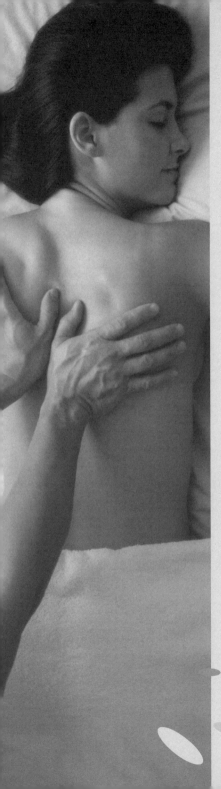

## 20

# Gold fingers

**Five minutes to spare? Try some self-massage: it's an inexpensive way to boost your circulation and kick-start your lymphatic drainage system.**

You can't underestimate the feel-good power of a great massage. It's relaxing but invigorating, and can alleviate all sorts of aches and pains.

Cellulite is a pain in the backside, and massage can help with that too. One study found that massage could boost circulation and stimulate the nerves that control blood flow to your organs. Another study  showed that deep mechanical massage really can help the appearance of cellulite.

Massage can help boost lymphatic drainage too – helping alleviate the fluid retention that can make you look puffy and bloated. And it has been shown to decrease levels of stress hormones, which are associated with weight gain. All good reasons to invest in a regular massage treatment.

If you have the funds to splash out on a salon massage, the best choice for cellulite sufferers is manual lymphatic drainage (MLD). This is a pleasant, deeply relaxing massage therapy, which is used to treat all sorts of health problems, from sprains, torn ligaments, sinusitis to rheumatoid arthritis. Beauty experts recommend it for fluid retention – it's a fantastic way to relieve tired, puffy eyes, and alleviate swollen ankles, that sort of thing. Plus it's thought to be an effective way to help heal wounds and minimise old scars.

> *Here's an idea for you...*
> **Very dry skin on your lower regions? Try massaging your legs and bottom with essential oil of sandalwood; it's a lovely lubricating oil that's very nourishing for dehydrated skin. It's also great for helping you sleep and for relieving anxiety. Add a drop or two to 15–20 ml carrier oil such as grapeseed or almond oil.**

During the first session, the therapist usually takes a thorough history – details of your health, lifestyle and concerns. Then you lie down, usually partially clothed, while the therapist uses a variety of gentle, rhythmic movements over your skin, in the direction of lymph flow. This gentle pumping action is thought to stimulate the lymphatic vessels, which helps removes waste products. By encouraging fluid loss, it can help improve the puffiness over the legs, bum and thighs. A course of six to ten treatments is usually recommended. Expect to pay about £30 a session.

Cheaper by far is a five-minute self-massage. All you need is some good oil or rich body moisturiser. Aim to incorporate a little routine into your morning or evening ablutions.

Massaging areas of your skin regularly – even for a few minutes a day – can help improve blood flow and lymph circulation, and moisturise your skin. When your skin is dry and dehydrated, cellulite appears far more noticeable.

Arm yourself with an aromatherapy-based oil or rich moisturising cream. Rub your hands together to warm the lotion/oil; this will make it easier to apply.

*Try another idea...*
**Saunas and steam baths can be wonderfully relaxing and purifying. Find out why it's worth getting hot and bothered in IDEA 48, *Some like it hot.***

If you find you tend to have more time in the evening, schedule your self-massage for bathtime, or bedtime. That way you can use it as a relaxation tool. Alternatively, try a few minutes self-massage after a workout to help soothe tired muscles.

Experts recommend spending a few minutes relaxing your muscles before you start. Sit or lie comfortably, and breathe in slowly for a count of four, then out to the count of four. Then rub your hands together to warm the lotion or aromatherapy oil.

Start with your thighs. Using a gentle but firm upwards stroke, work away from the knee. Always work upwards – toward the heart, so you're working with the circulation and lymph flow. Using loose fingers, gently 'knead' the thigh. Then place the palms of your hands flat on your buttocks and circle upwards and outwards, one hand on each buttock. Make sure you use long, slow, gentle movements. Next, massage your stomach. Use gentle circular movements – work in a circular position using the flats of your hands.

*Defining idea...*
**'Years wrinkle the skin, but to give up enthusiasm wrinkles the soul.'**
DOUGLAS MacARTHUR,
US general

Finally, move to your arms. Work your way upwards from your wrist to your shoulder, using a firm, but gentle, kneading motion. Then glide down your arm again to your wrist. Repeat several times on each arm.

## How did it go?

**Q: What about those massage tools you see in chemists and beauty stores? Are they any good?**

A: You can buy all sorts of massage aids – ones with rubber tips, wooden balls and even motorized massage heads. They're usually fairly cheap – say the cost of a bottle of wine – and can take your self-massage up a notch. But be careful not to be too energetic: over-zealous massaging can damage skin tissue. Alternatively, get someone to help you.

**Q: I quite like the idea of a series of manual lymphatic drainage. Any tips on salon etiquette?**

A: Taking off your clothes can be embarrassing – especially if you're a salon virgin – but remember you can always ask for a female masseuse when booking. If you do feel anxious during a treatment, you're not going to reap the full benefits, so make sure you tell your therapist you're not comfortable with taking everything off. She'll no doubt reassure you, and will tell you what to keep on so there'll be no surprises. A reputable practitioner will always leave the room as you undress. Then you can slip under a towel. He or she usually just uncovers bits of you at a time.

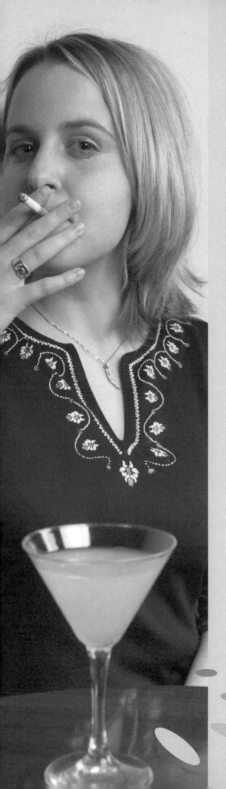

# 21

# Look at me, I'm Sandra Dee

**Cigarettes and alcohol contain toxins that wreak havoc with your skin. A dose of clean living might keep the dimples at bay.**

Smoking, drinking, late nights and wild living may be thrilling, but they're utterly bad news for thighs. Here's why.

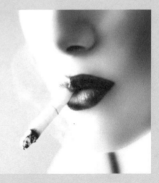

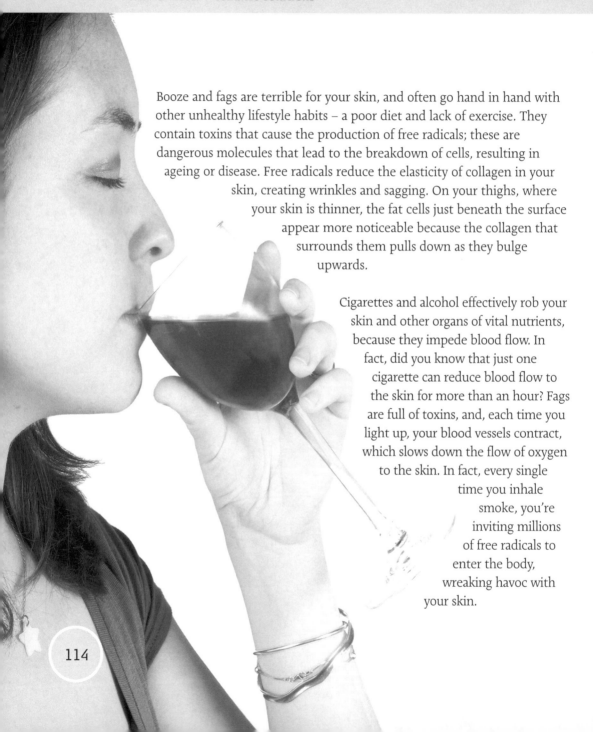

Booze and fags are terrible for your skin, and often go hand in hand with other unhealthy lifestyle habits – a poor diet and lack of exercise. They contain toxins that cause the production of free radicals; these are dangerous molecules that lead to the breakdown of cells, resulting in ageing or disease. Free radicals reduce the elasticity of collagen in your skin, creating wrinkles and sagging. On your thighs, where your skin is thinner, the fat cells just beneath the surface appear more noticeable because the collagen that surrounds them pulls down as they bulge upwards.

Cigarettes and alcohol effectively rob your skin and other organs of vital nutrients, because they impede blood flow. In fact, did you know that just one cigarette can reduce blood flow to the skin for more than an hour? Fags are full of toxins, and, each time you light up, your blood vessels contract, which slows down the flow of oxygen to the skin. In fact, every single time you inhale smoke, you're inviting millions of free radicals to enter the body, wreaking havoc with your skin.

And heavy drinking isn't much better. Experts warn us against binge drinking (that's anything over five units at a time), and drinking more than the recommended 14 units a week for women.

Long-term alcohol abuse can lead to liver and stomach problems, heart disease, cancer, plus it puts women at greater risk of sexual and physical attack.

At the very least it can cause weight gain and premature ageing – and make cellulite worse. That's because alcohol reduces your circulation, and causes dehydration, which robs the skin of moisture and vital nutrients. Plus when you're half cut, you're more likely to stuff your face with fish and chips, burgers, kebabs or a fatty curry, which encourages weight gain.

Alcohol causes an insulin surge, which causes blood sugar fluctuations – and this explains why you often wake up starving after a night out. That's when the prospect of a greasy fry-up is often so appealing. But that hangover breakfast can clock up as many as 1,000 calories.

Plus alcohol can disrupt your sleep, making you too tired for your cellulite-busting workout, and can also dent your self-control so you're more likely to be tempted by sugary sweets, junk food and treats.

Here's an idea
for you...
Want to lose weight but can't keep on the straight and narrow? Follow the 80/20 rule. As long as 80% of your food is nutritious, the other 20% doesn't have to be, because it's your eating habits over time that really govern your weight and health. Just think – that 20% could be fairy cakes, Swiss chocolates, spare ribs...mmmmm!

Defining idea...
'I cook with wine, sometimes I even add it to the food.'
W. C. FIELDS

On top of all that, alcohol calories can't be stored by the body, and they have to be used as they are consumed – this means that calories excess to requirements from other foods get stored as fat instead.

**What can you do:**

■ Limit your drinking – have alcohol-free days, and count those units religiously.

■ Stick to wine. Some experts say spirits are far worse for your skin, because they cause an inflammatory reaction there, which is potentially more damaging to your skin than the effects caused by wine.

■ Make it pricey stuff – you're more likely to savour instead of binge if you splashed out.

■ Never drink alcohol on an empty stomach. If you know you're going out that evening and will be drinking, try to include those drinks in your daily calorie allowance. Bear in mind that one small glass of red wine contains 85 calories, and a bottle of lager contains 130 calories.

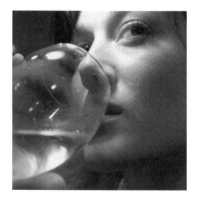

■ Resolve (again) to bin the cigarettes. Try your local smoking cessation programmes. Research says people who follow such programmes are four times more likely to succeed at giving up than those who go cold turkey.

*Try another idea...*

**Heading for the beach? Don't resign yourself to a wetsuit or kaftan. There are ways to flatter that behind. See how in IDEA 23, *With a thong in my heart.***

■ Hang out in no-smoking bars and restaurants. Spend more time with your non-smoking friends.

■ Review your social diary – swap those wild nights out for an exercise class, a run, or girly night in with a video, a face pack and nail varnish. Or start an evening class.

*Defining idea...*
**'One more drink and I'd have been under the host.'**
DOROTHY PARKER

## How did it go?

**Q: I'm afraid I just can't give up booze, however much I hate my cellulite. Have you got any tips to help me?**
A: Just try to drink in moderation – have alcohol-free days, and don't exceed the 14 units of alcohol a week (for women). And when you're drinking don't forget to drink plenty of water. Alcohol is dehydrating, and studies show that dehydration can slow your metabolism by up to 3%. Aim to have one glass of water for every alcoholic drink, and make sure you drink at least 1.5 litres a day.

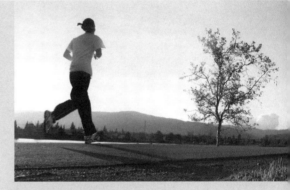

**Q: Is there anything else I can do to counteract the effects of my cigarette and chardonnay lifestyle?**
A: Take a daily antioxidant supplement which can help mop up the free radicals caused by alcohol and cigarette smoke – these free radicals precipitate ageing. Eat plenty of fresh fruits and veggies too – at least five portions a day. Beta-carotene is particularly important for smokers as it can help boost lung health. Get some fresh air daily and exercise regularly.

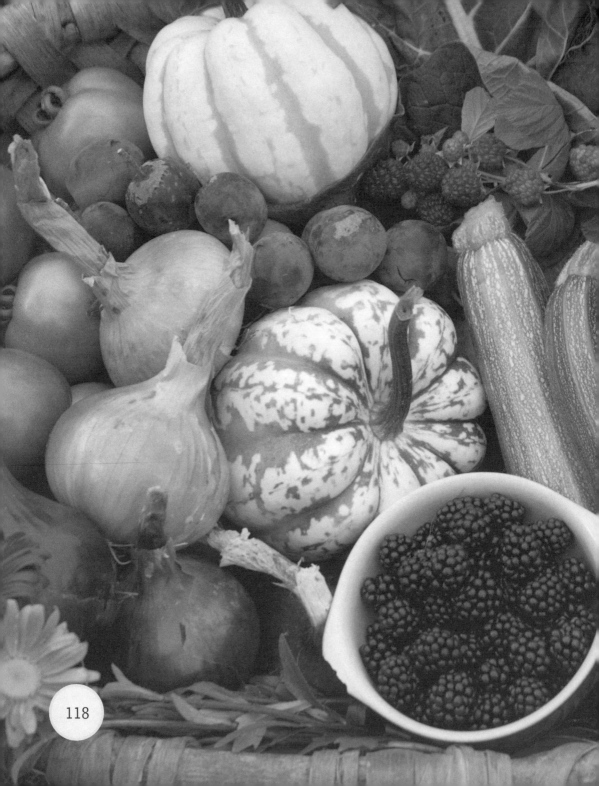

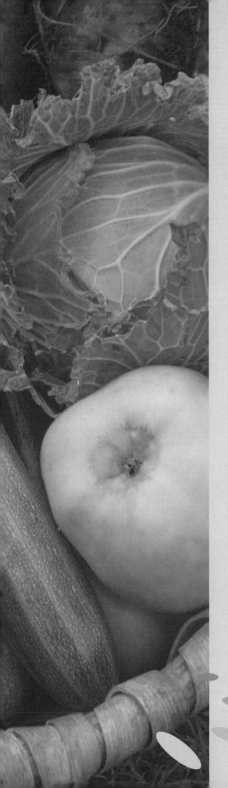

# 22

# Getting a skinful

**Certain foods contain skin-boosting nutrients that help keep the tissues between the fat cells supple, which can help minimise cellulite. Revamp your diet for smoother thighs.**

Some leading experts maintain that a firm ass is only as good as the skin that covers it.

Hydrating the skin and connective tissue that holds the fat in place, then, is the key to minimising cellulite. And the way to do that is by filling your body with the right foods.

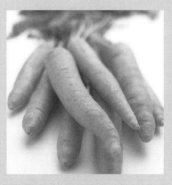

It makes sense, of course. You know yourself that eating nothing but junk takes its toll on your face, leading to pasty, dull, unruly skin. The same principle applies to your behind. If you're filling your face with processed foods, takeaways and skimping on fresh fruit, veg and lean proteins, it's little wonder that your tush looks lacklustre.

The good news is you can turn your skin around by choosing key nutrients in the right foods, ditching the wrong ones, and committing to a few new diet rules.

So here's what to put on your plate...

*Here's an idea for you...*

**Keep your tummy feeling fuller for longer by choosing the most filling foods, calorie per calorie. Studies on Satiety Index (SI) show that potatoes are twice as filling as grain bread, porridge or oatmeal is twice as filling as muesli, oranges are almost twice as filling as bananas and crackers are twice as filling as croissants!**

### Essential fatty acids

They're vital for the production of collagen, which helps keep your skin firm and those fat cells in place. They have a good anti-inflammatory action, and are great for improving the elasticity and texture of skin. Good sources include fish (especially salmon, tuna, mackerel), olive oil, flaxseed oil, nuts and seeds; these are all packed with omega-3 fatty acids which help control the lipids and fats in your body that can help skin stay soft and smooth. They're also rich in skin-friendly vitamin E. Brazil nuts contain the antioxidant selenium which helps fight free radicals. And try pumpkin seeds: they're another good source of omega-3 fatty acids, and contain vitamin E.

## Fruits and veggies

Fruit and veg are rich in antioxidants that help fight the free radicals that can lead to wrinkles. Free radicals not only cause cancer and heart disease, but can wreak havoc on skin by damaging your cell membranes and the connective tissues that support your skin.

*Try another idea...*

**If despite eating less and moving more, you're not shedding pounds and firming up, you may need some extra tips to boost your metabolism. Find out how in IDEA 14, *Top gear.***

Choose brightly coloured fruits and veg, make sure you eat at least five portions a day, and think variety. The brighter the fruit, the denser the concentration of nutrients – plus different coloured fruits contain different nutrients. So by choosing a variety of bright colours you ensure you're getting more nutrients than you would if you just ate a couple of apples. Berries are a great choice as they're bursting with antioxidants that help strengthen your blood capillaries. And they maintain healthy blood flow inside the connective tissues that support your skin.

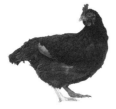

### Poultry

Turkey and chicken are great sources of lean protein, which is essential for making collagen. Poultry also contains an amino acid known as carnosine, which can help prevent wrinkles. Other good proteins to put on your plate include, eggs and soya products such as tofu, and drink skimmed milk. These are lean proteins so they're low in fat, but fill you up, and also contain skin-friendly amino acids.

### Spinach

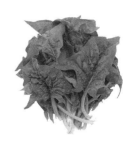

Popeye's favourite food is particularly rich in vitamin K, which is good for blood circulation, enabling nutrients to reach every cell. Spinach is also full of antioxidants, and is an anti-inflammatory, which helps protect cell walls. (Other good anti-inflammatories include broccoli, lettuce, beans, blackcurrants and olive oil.)

### Cruciferous veggies

Broccoli, cauliflower and cabbage are rich in antioxidants and fibre. They're also good for keeping your digestive system working properly and stimulating the liver, which helps removes waste and toxins from the body. When you lighten your toxic load, your skin looks better.

### Lecithin-rich foods

Lecithin is known for its ability to repair skin tissues. This nutrient is found in eggs, soya, cauliflower, spinach, lettuce and tomatoes.

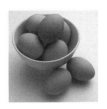

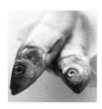

### B vitamins

You need B vitamins to provide energy, and for healthy digestion and skin. Good sources include dark leafy veg, low-fat dairy foods, fish, eggs, beans and wholegrains.

### Circulation-boosting foods

When your blood is circulating at optimum levels, it means that your cells – including your skin cells – are getting a regular supply of life-giving nutrients and oxygen. Good foods for circulation include onions, garlic, nuts, pumpkin seeds and fish.

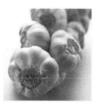

### Vitamin E-rich foods

Vitamin E is a powerful antioxidant that's good for healing and protecting skin as it plays an important role in cell maintenance. It's found in sweet potatoes, vegetable oils – especially soy and wheatgerm oil – sunflower seeds, wheatgerm, sweetcorn, cashews, almonds and peanuts. Avocados are another good source, and these handy fruits are also rich in vitamin C and healthy mono-unsaturated fats.

Defining idea...
*'Worthless people live only to eat and drink; people of worth eat and drink only to live.'* SOCRATES

## How did it go?

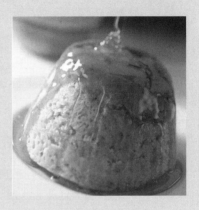

**Q: Are there any types of food I should be avoiding to beat cellulite?**

A: Aim to limit your intake of refined starches – such as cakes, biscuits and white bread – as these can make your skin puffy, dehydrated and prone to allergic reactions. Stick to wholegrains instead. Take sugary foods off the menu. These can raise your blood sugar, which interferes with the way the hormone insulin behaves. It's thought that if you flood your body with excess glucose, it causes collagen fibres to bunch up. The result? Loss of firmness and wrinkles. Sweeten foods with honey or fruit instead.

**Q: Are there any other foods I should steer clear of?**

A: Cut out the salty foods: these can cause fluid retention, which can make you look puffy and bloated. And also aim to swap red meat for chicken, turkey or fish and pulses, and avoid processed meats.

Defining idea...
**'When one has tasted watermelon, he knows what the angels eat.'**
MARK TWAIN

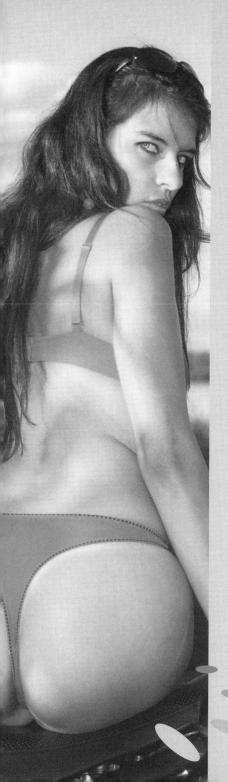

## 23

# With a thong in my heart

**Think before you disrobe. The right swimwear can flatter even the most dimply behind.**

Don't let a bit of cellulite ruin your beach days. With a bit of know-how you can still achieve St Tropez gorgeousness.

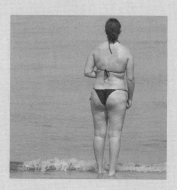

Remember that cellulite happens to the best of us. Pity those poor celebrities whose crinkly orange-peely bottoms are captured by the paparazzi as they frolic on exotic beaches, and are then plastered across the tabloids. Thankfully, most of us aren't subject to such scrutiny. Which means we can get away with a lot.

Basically there are four rules to surviving wearing very little when you have cellulite. Follow them, and you can still get almost-naked with confidence.

> Here's an idea
> for you...
> **Capitalise on the exotic fresh fruits on offer at your holiday buffet. Fill your plate with yummy papaya and pineapple – they contain a compound called bromelain, which can help beat bloating.**

## 1. Rebalance

Cellulite often, but not always, goes hand in hand with saddlebag thighs and a pear-shaped body. The first step, then, is to rebalance your silhouette. Always go for the mix-and-match option of bikinis so your itsy-bitsy will actually fit; otherwise, unless you're a perfect Sophia Loren–style hour-glass, something will gape or pull unflatteringly over your flesh. This will make the dimples more noticeable.

- Don't be tempted to grab a cheap string bikini at the airport – particularly without trying it on. If you're going somewhere hot, chances are you'll be living in it for two weeks, so invest appropriately. It's worth getting separates that flatter your figure and make you feel so much more confident on the beach – particularly if you're top or bottom heavy. Good investment brands are Jets or Melissa Odabash.

- Big bottom? Opt for flippy skirt bottoms – they're great for camouflaging thick cellulitey thighs.

- String ties are actually more flattering than too-tight cuts that make hips and thighs bulge over the top.

- To minimise a curvaceous bum, try a dark solid colour on the bottom and put the colour and pattern on top. Balance out a flat chest with a bandeau-style bikini.

*Try another idea...*
**Don't let your cellulite get you down. Men rarely notice it, we've found. In IDEA 32, *Billy Liar?*, you can discover what they're really thinking about when they see you naked.**

## 2. Disguise

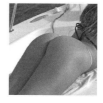

- Fake tan is a must. Get a salon treatment or do a DIY job before you hit the sun. Look for suntan cream with fake tan base and pack an aftersun with a tan prolonger. The browner those cheeks look, the smoother they'll appear.

- Don't cross your legs on the beach bar stool – it squishes the cellulite and makes it look worse. Sit strategically on your sunbed or beach towel; only the under-14s (that's age and dress size) should actually sit up straight on the beach – never sit upright or your tummy will look like a concertina. Instead, lean back on your elbows, with your legs stretched out, looking relaxed and casual.

- Watch the pattern on your swimwear. Large motifs tend to make you look fleshier than you are, so make sure the motif is smaller than your fist. Tankinis are brilliant for disguising cellulitey or bulgy midriffs or waists. Look for swimwear with clever control panels which lift your bum and your bust.

127

## 3. Enhance

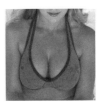

■ Draw attention from your lower regions and put your other assets on display.

■ Give yourself a great pre-bikini shape up by applying some bust-firming creams. The results tend to be temporary but they can help firm up a sagging décolletage and boost elasticity. Elemis and Thalgo have some great bust- and body-firmers.

■ Draw more attention to your boobs with padded bras, frilly bits, bright colours horizontal stripes, or try underwired shapes with bows or flowers for extra oomph.

■ If you have monster cellulite avoid those white swimsuits, which are often more than revealing when wet. Instead stick to black, or, if you've achieved a gorgeous bronzed body, flirt with tangerine, petrol blue or emerald green, which all look great with a tan.

> ### Defining idea...
> *'A girl in a bikini is like having a loaded pistol on your coffee table – there's nothing wrong with them, but it's hard to stop thinking about it'.*
> GARRISON KEILLOR

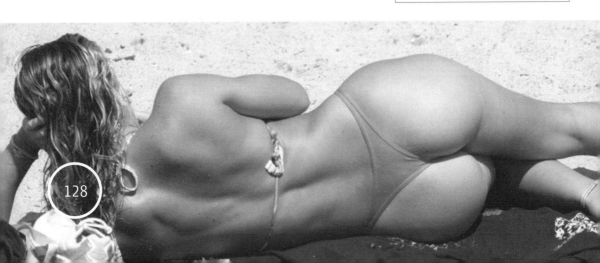

## 4. Distract

- Accessories are a great way to distract the eye from the bits you don't want to see. Invest in a flowing kaftan (Elizabeth Hurley's beach range is a godsend to cellulite sufferers), stylish beach bag, and dainty jewellery. One really special piece that sets off a beach outfit and makes you feel gorgeous and is worth the investment. Bangles or corals can be bargain buys.

- Stick to summer cottons or light linens that won't hug your curvy bits too unforgivingly.

- A pair of wedge-soled sandals or espadrilles gives you extra inches to make you feel leggy and willowy – and instantly more attractive.

- Paint your toenails beautifully, blow dry your hair or pin up tendrils for water-baby glamour.

- Make sure your skin looks baby soft. Don't undress without attending to all those beach body ablutions – hair removal on legs and bikini line, etc.

> Defining idea...
> **'An optimist is a girl who mistakes a bulge for a curve.'**
> RING LARDNER, writer

## How did it go?

**Q: OK, I haven't dieted or exercised, but I'm heading to the sun for an impromptu beach weekend. What can I wear to disguise a dimply tummy?**

A: Make sure you pack a lovely floaty kaftan and great swimsuit. Then, if you're after quickie solutions, head to the duty-free shop and pop a toning product in your bag. Some of these toners are formulated specifically for your tummy area, and usually contain skin-firming ingredients that act as a kind of girdle for your midriff. Plus they're imbued with ingredients to help boost circulation to improve skin tone. Best ones include Biotherm Abdo Choc, Clarins Total Body Lift, L'Oreal Sculpt Up.

**Q: My stomach's became flabby after having kids. What are the best swimwear styles to opt for to disguise the bulges?**

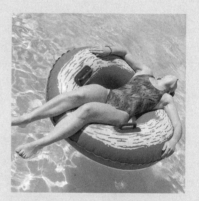

A: If you're happier in a two piece, you can hide a bulging tummy with a tankini – they have built-in support to cover a bulging tum – or high-cut bikini bottoms that come higher over your tummy. Belted bottoms help create a waist and make you look slimmer round the middle.

# 24

# The big easy

**Beware! Quickie crash diets may make cellulite worse. Small, simple weight-loss habits have longer-lasting effects.**

If you've ever tried a crash diet or 'fasted' to get into that little dress, you'll know that restricting your calorie intake just doesn't pay in the long term.

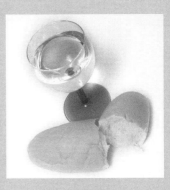

Nutrition experts are united in the condemnation of crash diets, which usually involve eating fewer than 1000 calories a day. OK, these diets may help you drop a few pounds sharpish, but they're really not going to transform your body for very long. And they're likely to make cellulite worse. Here's why.

Firstly, following a crash diet usually means you miss out on nutrients. If you stick to one of those bizarre nothing-but-bread-and-water, or boiled-egg-only diets, or grapefruit fasts, you're not going to be getting all the protein, carbohydrates, healthy fats, and vitamins and minerals you need to stay healthy – and to maintain healthy skin.

The bottom line is if you deprive your body of nutrients, your skin will suffer. If your skin loses some of its elasticity, the collagen fibres that hold the fat pockets in place won't be so springy. As a result, the fat that causes those dimples will appear more pronounced.

Secondly, long-term fasting or crash dieting can affect your metabolic rate, which drops when you're not eating because your body tries to conserve energy when it's not getting enough food. And this means that when you do start eating normally again (and who can honestly stay on a crash diet for any length of time?) you'll gain weight.

Repeated yo-yo crash dieting also makes cellulite worse because it tends to cause loss of muscle tissue. Studies show that severe crash dieting actually depletes more lean tissue than slow dieting does. Muscle not only helps you burn more calories, but it's great for keeping cellulite at bay because it fills your skin out more and helps keep it taut. Fat, on the other hand, takes up more space so it bulges out, making cellulite worse.

Crash diets don't encourage good, sensible eating habits, either, which are the key to long-term weight loss. If you really want to lose weight and shift cellulite, you need to create small calorie deficits in your diet, and to take more exercise.

Exercise really is crucial: it boosts your metabolic rate, and builds muscle. In fact, one study showed that people who didn't diet but took more exercise lost on average about 3 kg a year.

> *Try another idea...*
> **Dry skin-brushing takes a few minutes a day, and you'll see the benefits almost immediately. Find out more in IDEA 4, *Give it the brush-off*.**

133

Convinced yet? Time to throw away that faddy diet book and instead adopt a few sensible weight-loss habits. Try these tricks:

- Keep a diary of what you've been eating. In one study, people who 'self-monitored' lost 64% more weight than those who didn't – *and* maintained the weight loss three months later.

- Limit the booze – stick to a glass a night or a pricier bottle once or twice a week.

- Savour food – make it an occasion, so you're relishing each bite. Stop eating on the run, and ban munching in front of the telly.

- Eat the lowest-calorie foods on your plate first – usually the vegetables or salad. Then eat the next lowest-calorie food. Ending with the highest-calorie food means you may be too full to finish it – plus you'll have eaten all your greens.

- Make healthier choices at business lunches – skip the starters or have two starters rather than a starter and a main course.

- Get healthier snacks – flapjacks instead of eclairs, skimmed milk cappuccinos instead of full-fat lattes.

- Cut down on takeaways or fatty convenience foods. Invest in low-fat microwave meals, frozen or microwaveable veggies, even packet noodles for healthy last-minute suppers.

- Never shop when you're hungry, and always plan your meals.

- Had a binge day? The day after try to cut 200–500 calories from your daily calorie allowance to compensate. Or exercise for an extra 20 or 30 minutes

- Start reading labels on food packets.

- Only eat when you're really hungry. Ask yourself how hungry you are on a scale of zero to ten – if it's six or less, do something else instead!

- Make lunch the biggest meal of the day; your metabolism is more efficient then.

- Exercise, exercise, exercise!

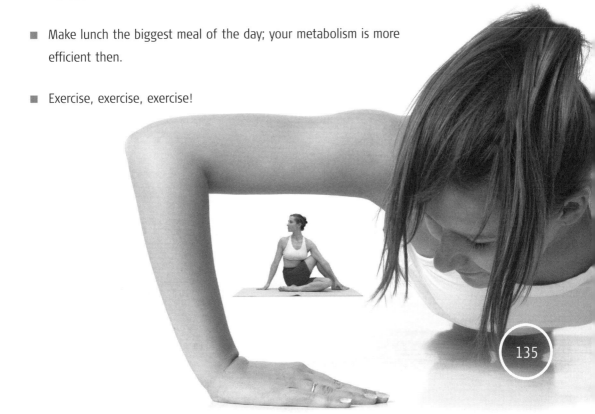

135

# How did it go?

**Q: I'm not someone who snacks between meals, but I do tend to eat a lot at mealtimes. How can I curb my appetite?**

A: New studies show that eating a small apple or pear before your meals, while following a low-calorie diet, can help you lose more weight. Apparently these fruits are great at filling you up, which means you end up eating less at mealtimes. Eating slowly and drinking a glass of water before you sit at the table should help too.

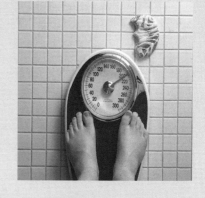

**Q: How can I stop craving my favourite, high-calorie foods?**

A: Stop counting calories, and take things off the forbidden list. When you're eating out, instead of choosing the dish with the lowest number of calories, just go ahead and order what you fancy. Just eat a bit of it, or half of it so you feel you've indulged without going overboard. Try sticking to the 10% sweets rule (that's 200 calories if your intake is about 2000 calories a day). If you must, eat something sweet with each meal: a light mousse, frozen yoghurt, an ice-lolly, a big fruit salad with ice-cream – or a bag of sweets for pudding. A small treat may keep you on track.

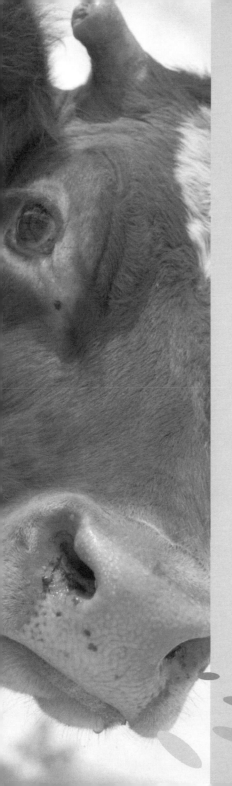

# 25

# Food of the gods (and goddesses)

**Protein helps build muscles, boosts your metabolism, fills you up. Cellulite hates it!**

'Get plenty of protein into your diet' sounds like the advice dispensed to burly bodybuilders. But it could hold the key to shifting your cellulite.

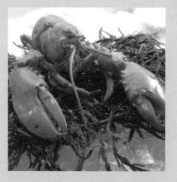

**Protein is a cellulite-sufferer's friend for several reasons.**

Firstly, because it can help you lose weight. Many experts believe that fat – plain, old fat – is the real cause of cellulite. More precisely, they say that cellulite is caused by pockets of fat bulging out from beneath your skin. And even if you're slim elsewhere, you probably store fat on your bottom and thighs (most women do), and that's where cellulite lurks. So shift some fat, and you'll shift some cellulite.

Protein helps you lose pounds because it helps keep your blood sugar levels steady, which means you stay feeling fuller for longer. It also helps prevent sugar cravings, so you'll be less likely to be tempted by that ice-cream sundae, cake or chocolate bar.

Secondly, protein also contains important amino acids that help produce fresh collagen, so it's good for your skin – whether it's on your face or your behind. Keeping your skin in great condition means your cellulite is less noticeable.

Protein also helps build muscle. By increasing your muscle mass, you'll boost your metabolic rate, and your body will become more efficient at burning off calories.

*Here's an idea for you...*

Want a simple, low-calorie appetite suppressant? Try a snack of hummous and an oatcake or crispbread. It's an instant energy booster, and a great way to rebalance your blood sugar levels and fill you up till supper time.

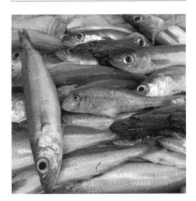

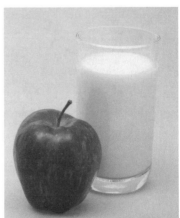

Experts also say that proteins contain a substance called albumin, which helps absorb excess fluid in your tissues. Water retention around the thighs and bottom is another oft-quoted cause of cellulite. So if you tend to retain water, aim to eat optimum amounts of lean protein to help reduce water retention.

*Try another idea...*

**Who knew a stressed mind can lead to dimply thighs? Find out why and how to chill out – pronto. See IDEA 19, *The big chill*.**

Oh, and protein's also good for your brain function too. And if you eat enough of it, it'll make you so sharp-witted, cerebral and brilliant that no one will notice your cellulite anyway.

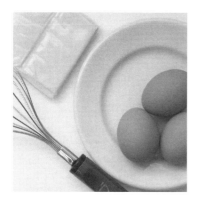

## So how much protein should I be eating exactly?

About 15–20% of your diet should come from proteins and we should aim to eat three portions a day. Women need about 45 g each day. If you consume a 2,000 calories-per-day diet, roughly 300 of those calories should come from protein. Use your plate as a gauge: divide it into three and imagine filling about a third with protein foods such as turkey, cottage cheese, fish and nuts.

Recent studies have shown that just by increasing your daily intake of protein to 25–30% you can lose several kilos. But don't go overboard. High-protein diets may have been all the rage this millennium, but they come with heavy warnings from nutritionists as excessive intakes of protein can have adverse effects on your kidneys, your bones and your breath!

So if you want to increase your protein intake, make sure it doesn't exceed 30% of your overall dietary intake. And also make sure you eat plenty of calcium-rich foods such as cottage cheese and yoghurt, as some research suggests that diets rich in protein may prevent calcium loss from the bones.

## What's a portion?

A portion is about the size of your fist. That's equivalent to 25 g of nuts, about 50–75 g cooked lean meat, fish or poultry, one egg or 100 g cooked beans.

Here's a guide to how much protein you get in different food sources:

| | |
|---|---|
| 155 g lean rump steak | 44 g protein |
| 85 g lean roast chicken | 26 g protein |
| 130 g grilled cod steak | 27 g protein |
| boiled egg | 8 g protein |
| 1 litre semi-skimmed milk | 33 g protein |
| 150 g low-fat yoghurt | 7 g protein |
| 40 g cheddar cheese | 10 g protein |
| 200 g tin baked beans | 10 g protein |
| 30 g peanuts | 7 g protein |

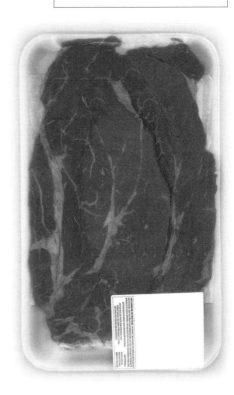

*Defining idea...*

'**Vegetables are interesting but lack a sense of purpose when unaccompanied by a good cut of meat.**'
FRAN LEBOWITZ, American writer

# Mix 'n' match your proteins

- **Amino acids** Animal proteins such as meat, poultry, fish and dairy produce contain all the eight essential amino acids your body needs, but plant proteins (nuts, pulses, grains and seeds) lack some of these, so veggies and vegans should make sure they eat a variety of different protein sources each day.

- **Calcium** Dairy proteins – yoghurt, milk and cheese are the obvious sources.

- **Omega-3 fatty acids** Fish – particularly salmon, tuna, herring, sardines, mackerel and trout – is rich in these fatty acids, which are good for your skin.

- **Fibre and vitamins** Beans are a great source of low-fat protein, and are also rich in fibre and B vitamins. Nuts and seeds are rich in protein, fibre, minerals and vitamin E. Prawns are rich in the antioxidant selenium, vitamin B12 for healthy blood, and iodine for healthy thyroid function, plus they're a tasty low-fat source of protein.

# Yo Soya!

Soya products such as tofu are the only plant-based food equivalent to animal products in terms of protein quality. They're packed with complex carbs and B vitamins, zinc, potassium, magnesium and iron. They're also loaded with fibre and are rich in calcium. Soya products also contain isoflavones, which may protect you from certain cancers.

# How did it go?

**Q: What's the best form of protein to keep the dimples down?**

A: A healthy variety of sources is the best advice. But when it comes to keeping skin looking good and your weight down (which are both crucial for beating cellulite), oily fish is a top choice. It's low in calories, but rich in omega-3 fatty acids: these repair skin and help keep it elastic and firm.

**Q: Should I avoid red meat? Is it bad for my cellulite?**

A: Depends. Lean red meat is a great source of iron and zinc, and B vitamins, which are important for energy and growth. But if you eat lots of fatty red meat and processed foods such as sausages and bacon, you'll almost certainly gain weight, and therefore make your cellulite worse. In fact one recent study found that vegetarians, vegans or semi-vegetarians were less likely to be obese than meat eaters. But you don't have to give up red meat completely. Eat it once a week, and the rest of the time stick to low-fat proteins such as skinless chicken, beans, nuts or fish.

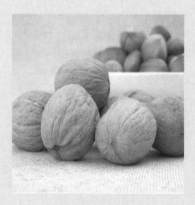 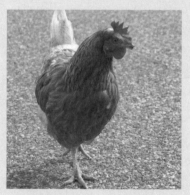

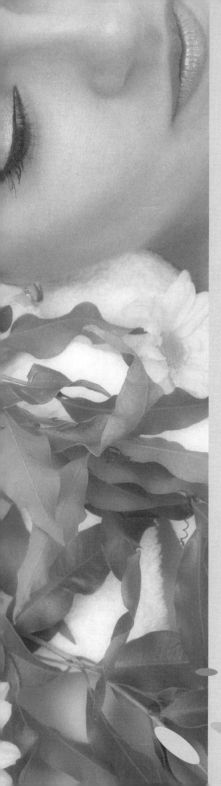

# 26

# Scents of a woman

**Natural remedies, essential oils and aromatherapy treatments can help reduce cellulite.**

Most us think of aromatherapy as a great solution to chronic stress — it conjures lovely images of flopping down in a therapy room while some nimble-fingered practitioner drops beautiful smelling oils on our back and gets to work undoing those knots.

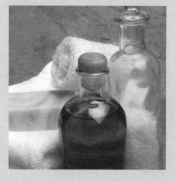

But essential oils have farther-reaching powers. As well as helping a variety of problems from anxiety to headaches, acne to irregular periods and insomnia, aromatherapy can also be a great ally in the fight against cellulite.

For example, certain essential oils have therapeutic properties which can help regulate your hormones (oestrogen is thought to be a contributing factor both to cellulite and to being overweight); others are great for the skin, and some have effective diuretic qualities so they can help beat water retention, which many of us blame for our bulgy thighs.

So whether you're happier putting your bottom in an aromatherapist's hands, or you fancy some DIY cellulite busting, here's your guide to which essential oils can do what.

**Note:** *Some essential oils shouldn't be used during pregnancy or with certain medical conditions, so always check with a qualified practitioner.*

Here's an idea
for you...
**Try a daily vitamin E supplement. It is great for your skin, plus a lack of vitamin E has been found to cause fluid retention. Or try upping your intake of vitamin E in dietary forms – with olive oil, nuts, seeds or brown rice.**

# The Fluid fighters

These can help boost your lymphatic drainage system and alleviate the water retention, which is thought to contribute to cellulite.

**Try another idea...**

Feeling bloated? Water retention can make your tummy protrude and your bottom dimple. Try changing your diet with IDEA 51, *The winds of change.*

- **Rosemary** is known for its refreshing, diuretic and purifying qualities, and may help beat water retention. (Avoid during pregnancy, if you're epileptic or have high blood pressure.)

- **Sweet fennel** has a cleansing and tonic action, particularly good for helping you purify your insides after overindulging in food! It's good for your digestive system and has diuretic properties so it can help with water retention. Smells lovely and aniseedy. (Don't use when pregnant or if you suffer from epilepsy.)

- **Atlas cedarwood** – this dry-woody smelling oil has a diuretic action, so it can help alleviate fluid retention and is thought to encourage the lymphatic drainage. Aromatherapists also say it can help stimulate the breakdown of fats. (Avoid during pregnancy.)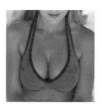

- **Grapefruit** is known to be a lymphatic stimulant, so it may help with fluid retention. It has a stimulating effect on bile, so is thought to help boost fat digestion. Tangy, refreshing scent.

- **Patchouli** – this exotic oil has a strong spicy smell and is known for its diuretic properties, so could help with fluid retention.

- **Geranium** has a lovely sweet smell. It's a great circulation booster and is good for fluid retention too.

- **Cypress** – this refreshing fragrance is known for its regulating effects on the body's fluids. Plus it's good for your circulation.

- **Juniper** is a detoxifier. It's good for relieving fluid retention, and can be stimulating and refreshing.

## The Skin enhancers

Cellulite looks worse when the skin is dehydrated or as you age and lose that plump firmness. The following can help boost your skin health:

- **Rosemary** is an energising, stimulating oil with astringent properties – it's believed to be useful in helping to tighten sagging skin on backs of legs, bottom and thighs.

- **Grapefruit** is rich in vitamin C, a good antioxidant, so it's good nourishment for your skin and aids repair.

- **Patchouli** is healing and is thought to encourage the growth of new skin cells.

- **Cypress** can help rebalance fluid loss and is great for rehydrating dry skin on bottoms and thighs.

- **Sweet fennel** has a tonic action which can help tone saggy, wrinkly skin.

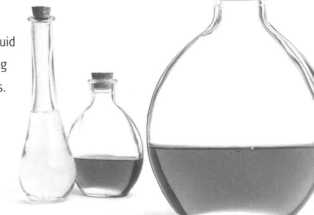

## The hormone rebalancers

The hormone oestrogen is linked with cellulite: certain oils are said to help normalise out-of-kilter hormone levels which are associated with weight gain.

- **Cypress** is known for its ability to help balance female hormone levels.

- **Sweet fennel** has a natural oestrogen content so may have a positive effect on your oestrogen levels.

## How to use your essential oils

- Try self-massage. You'll moisturise your cellulitey areas at the same time and your skin will look instantly smoother and plumper. Mix six drops of essential oils with about 3–4 tsp (15–20 ml) of carrier oil such as sweet almond oil or grapeseed oil. (Don't use essential oils neat on the skin as they can cause irritation.)

- Bathe in them. Add four to six drops to warm water. Adding milk or vodka can help disperse the oils.

- Pop them on a tissue and smell them.

- Try burning them in a diffuser and inhale the scent.

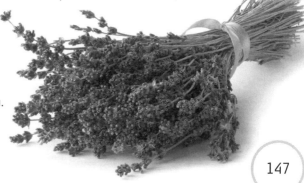

# How did it go?

### Q: My cellulite has become worse since I've gained weight. Can you suggest any natural appetite suppressants?

A: Aromatherapists say that essential oils containing patchouli can dull the appetite. Try sprinkling it on a tissue or burn it in a diffuser during mealtimes. You may find you end up eating less, and you'll smell nicer too! Juniper is a good essential oil as it helps regulate the appetite – useful if haphazard munching is making you chubby.

### Q: Can you suggest any easy essential oil recipes I can whip up myself?

A: Try a home-made anti-cellulite massage oil. Mix together 15 ml (1 tbsp) almond oil, 2 drops wheatgerm oil, 8 drops cumin oil, 2–3 drops orange or lemon oil. Use it after a bath or shower to massage your legs, thighs and tummy areas. Remember some essential oils aren't recommended during pregnancy or with some health conditions. Check with a qualified practitioner.

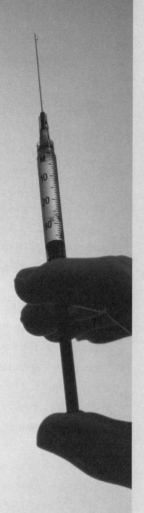

# 27

# The next big thing?

**A new treatment has been discovered that could actually destroy fat cells in your cellulite-prone areas – permanently.**

Injecting carbon dioxide directly into the layer of cellulite under the skin can break through cell walls and liquefy the fat, ready for elimination from the body. So will you be one of the first to try it?

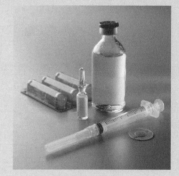

In one of the most innovative skin-care developments for a long time, doctors in Italy recently found that carbon dioxide injections that were used to successfully

149

treat leg ulcers could also have an effect on cellulite. Now this promising new treatment is arriving in the UK, with the first salons set to offer the injections in March 2006.

The injections go deeper into the skin than the other main anti-cellulite treatment involving injections, mesotherapy, right down to the fat layer containing all those pesky lumps and bumps we hate so much. But why carbon dioxide? Because it can apparently kill off fat cells in the areas targeted specifically by the injections. Carbon dioxide can also help widen the capillaries in the skin tissue, resulting in better blood flow and more oxygen and nutrients being delivered to the skin. This may also result in less fluid between the cells, which means firmer skin.

The procedure seems surprisingly straightforward compared to some other technological cellulite treatments. Using a micro-fine needle, the cellulite-sufferer is given several injections, depending on the size of the area being treated, of purified, medically approved carbon dioxide gas. A narrow tube links the needle with a cylinder storing the gas, which in turn is attached to a machine. The machine filters the gas to medical standards and warms it up – cold gas would feel very painful when injected.

*Here's an idea for you...*

OK, so you've got cellulite, but how bad is it really? Try the 'pinch test' right now to see what stage yours is at. Put your thumbs and forefingers in each corner of a square of skin where you think the dimply stuff is. Then squeeze gently. If your bumps are pretty evenly spaced, your cellulite hasn't yet reached an advanced stage. So don't eat junk, drink 6–8 glasses of water a day and get your running shoes on two or three times a week. Check it again after six weeks – you may be pleasantly surprised.

Talking of pain, yes, there is an 'element of discomfort' involved in this treatment (what do you expect, miracles?). How much discomfort depends on your personal pain threshold but, helpfully, the manufacturers of the machines say that treatment can be stopped at any time. If all this is sounding a bit like torture, apparently the sensation lessens with each session, and in any case – a big plus – the whole business is over in minutes.

*Try another idea...*

**A powerful plant used in folk medicine for centuries has been shown to help in the battle of the bulging thighs. What is it, where do you find it, and how do you take it? Turn to IDEA 50, *Grass roots*, to find out.**

Reports from Italy have revealed varied, but some quite impressive, results, with smoother skin and less obvious dimples. Tests have involved just treating one leg and comparing it with the untreated one. And interestingly, trials in Italy were done with women who were not following a weight-loss diet or exercise regime. This gives a clearer picture of the treatment's effectiveness. Often, when someone's starting a course of treatment plus a new healthy eating plan and exercise, it's hard to tell what is really causing any cellulite reduction.

For the best results, a course of about 12–15 treatment sessions is recommended, ideally two per week. So you have to devote a bit of time to this over a couple of months. Obviously it's going to help if you've saved up some money for this little lot, though carbon dioxide is actually pretty cheap, and as the treatment doesn't take that long, salons shouldn't be charging huge amounts. The cost should be less than, say, endermologie treatments, which involve an expensive machine and more time.

*Defining idea...*

*'New ideas pass through three periods:*
*– It can't be done.*
*– It probably can be done, but it's not worth doing.*
*– I knew it was a good idea all along!'*
ARTHUR C. CLARKE

You should be able to see improvements about halfway through the schedule. The big question: is it permanent or is it temporary? To date, most salon cellulite treatments veer more towards the temporary, with regular top-up sessions needed to 'keep up appearances'.

If early reports are to be believed, carbon dioxide therapy has the potential to be long term. For a start, the body has a finite number of fat cells, and if you are killing some of them off, they're gone for good. Whether it's long term or not does, however, depend on you too. If you stick to your ideal weight and a healthy diet that won't encourage cellulite formation, plus the usual health advice such as drinking plenty of water, then, theoretically at least, the dimples shouldn't return.

## How did it go?

**Q: Isn't carbon dioxide toxic? Are you sure this treatment is safe?**
A: Carbon dioxide is created naturally in the body – we breathe it out through our lungs – and carbon dioxide therapy is used to treat certain medical conditions. It's carbon monoxide that's the poisonous one (remember those science lessons?). A study published in the *Aesthetic Plastic Surgery Journal* reported no serious side effects for carbon dioxide therapy, and as far as we can tell this treatment appears to be safe.

**Q: I'm not too sure about gas being injected under my skin. Where does the gas go?**
A: Good question. Apparently the gas can make bubbles form beneath the skin during this treatment, which can look a bit alarming to say the least. But the bubbles disappear within a few minutes as the gas disperses under the skin, so there shouldn't be too much danger of ending up looking like an Aero bar.

# 28

# Tomorrow's world

**Send in the boffins: it's time for science to come to the rescue. Here's how the latest high-tech treatments can help zap cellulite away.**

We could all do with a bit of sci-fi wizardry to help smooth crinkly thighs. After all, what's science for? Keep up to speed on the latest gizmos.

Laser treatments used to be offered to cellulite sufferers until the arrival of endermologie, the machine-based massage therapy and one of the very few cellulite treatments to get hard-to-come-by approval from the US Food and Drug Administration (FDA). At that time, clinics and salons tended to stop doing laser and switched instead to endermologie, which gave better results.

But it's a different story now. Endermologie is still a favoured cellulite-buster, but the next generation of treatments has arrived. These have two, if not three, different elements, often including both endermologie and laser technology, with maybe a heat source, such as radiofrequency, thrown in. In the race to find ever more effective treatments, new therapies with tech-y names keep appearing, many of which overlap confusingly with one another. It's enough to make you pine for the days when all you had to choose from was a good old body-brush or a pot of cream (well, almost)!

But it's worth checking out these new therapies, because some serious money and research is going into the quest for the holy grail of cellulite treatments, and out there somewhere could be the one that works for you. That said, don't swallow everything you read in brochures or on company websites –and it's best not to expect miracles, however high-tech the treatment sounds.

Here's an idea
for you...
**Don't check your cellulite in the bathroom mirror. Bathroom lighting is often bright and harsh – well that's fine when you're tweezering your eyebrows or putting your contact lenses in. But who the heck is going to see you in that light except for you? So boost your confidence and check out your thighs in another mirror – yep, even if you have to stand on the dining-room table under that chandelier...**

One new treatment, known as Velasmooth, was developed in the USA and has already been given FDA approval. It uses a combination of massage rollers and vacuum sucking of the dimply fat (like endermologie) to help break fatty deposits down, and infrared light and radiofrequency (a bit like microwave technology). The idea is that warming up the fat will soften it and make it easier to disperse. Whatever you make of being partly cooked, vacuumed and pummelled – and some of the more sensitive among you might not like it much at all – so far much of the photographic evidence of the results coupled with first-hand experience make it look worth a try. A big plus seems to be that, as long as you can commit to having enough treatments in a fairly short space of time, results can be pretty rapid.

Try another idea...
**No time to lose and prepared to spend, spend, spend? Endomeso, the Rolls Royce of cellulite treatments, could be for you. Turn to IDEA 31,** *Salon selectives.*

Be warned, though, that with this, and other machine-dependent treatments, you may have to keep going back for more to keep your thighs looking good – a bit like botox for the forehead or facial lines, or collagen for plumping up lips.

# What's up next?

One of the top laser development companies, previously known for using laser technology to zap acne, reduce age spots and remove tattoos, is launching a new variation on cellulite zapping in time for summer 2006. Called Bio-cellulate, this

Defining idea...
*'Any sufficiently advanced technology is indistinguishable from magic.'*
ARTHUR C. CLARKE

one combines deep endermologie massage with infrared laser therapy, and research and trial results are described as 'exciting'.

Word from the moles in the white coats is that a million dollars has been spent on MRI scanners that can measure the depth of fat deposits, so that cellulite layers beneath the skin can be more easily targeted. And follow-up results on testers apparently show that thighs can remain smoother for six or even twelve months without their owners having to resort to more treatment – provided healthy lifestyle rules are followed, of course.

One other reason these high-tech, rapid-result treatments might be worth investing in is if you have a special event in mind. A beach wedding maybe (whether your own or someone else's), a holiday with someone you hope might fall in love with your fabulous figure (of course he's already fallen in love with your bubbly personality and superior mind), or a night of romance when you might be giving your best underwear an airing. Enjoy!

## How did it go?

**Q: I'm dying to try some of this new stuff. But am I going to have to take out a bank loan first?**

A: Possibly. Well, they loan money for home improvements, so why not bottom improvements? Or how about marrying the man in the white coat who's got the keys to the cellulite-zapping treatment room? Seriously, some of these therapies can get expensive, especially when you start layering all these new technologies together. That glossy machinery doesn't come cheap, so all the more reason to choose carefully. See if you can talk to other cellulite sufferers who've had a full course of treatment and find out what difference it has made to them before you commit to anything costly.

**Q: What about my love handles? I'm not particularly overweight but as well as cellulite I've got fatty bits above my hips that I can't seem to shift. Will these fancy treatments do the trick?**

A: Some of these treatments might be worth a try if you've got persistent fatty deposits in specific areas, as the word is they can work. Investigate the ones that claim to 'sculpt' the body as well as do battle with cellulite. Good luck – and be careful out there!

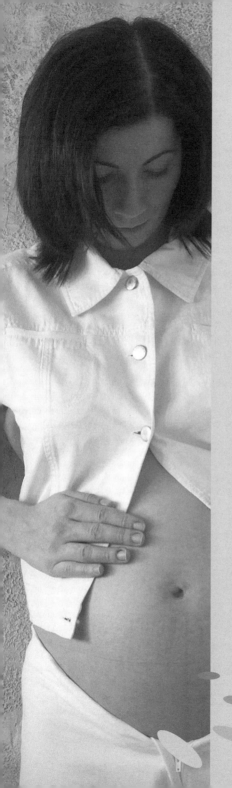

# 29

# Mother's ruin

**Cellulite often comes down to genetics. Take our test – then follow the best strategies to reverse your leg-acy.**

Yes, you can inherit cellulite. But though it might be just as hard to shift as the antique trunk in the attic, you're not necessarily stuck with it.

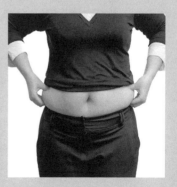

157

# Take the gene test

**1.** Is your mother the same body shape as you, and are you both heavier around the bottom than the top? Stand side by side in front of a mirror and, regardless of weight or age, you'll get a good idea.

**2.** Go back another generation and look at those lovely old photos of your granny when she was young. Recognise that good old family pear shape?

**3.** Do you get very cold hands and feet – and does your mother too?

**4.** Do you have fine or 'thin' skin like your mother, the type that allows veins to show through more easily?

The more 'yes' answers you gave to these questions, the more likely it is that your cellulite is in your genes. Take your body shape. You might think you look totally different to your mother, but that may have more to do with style and clothes than what's underneath them. We can trim and hone as much as we like, but our basic body shape remains the same from the day we are born. It's genetics that decides, where we're going to store our fat, and if that's around our thighs or backside – the classic pear shape – we're more likely to develop cellulite.

There's no shortage of experts who believe that sluggish circulation in the smallest blood vessels contributes to cellulite. The skin can't be at its healthiest if it doesn't get a good supply of oxygen and nutrients via the blood. One of the signs of poor circulation is slow-healing bruises, as well as cold hands and feet. If your fingers go white and numb in chilly weather, like your mother's, chances are you share the slow-circulation gene.

Are you thick skinned or thin skinned? Skin type varies from one woman to the next, and thinner skins allow the 'cellulite layer' – the bumpy fat tissues under the skin – to be seen more easily.

You might well have inherited all of this lot (thanks, mum!). That doesn't mean diet, exercise and other cellulite-busting ideas won't help, it's just that if your mother is cellulite prone and so are you, then it's going to be harder to shift than, say, someone who has the dreaded dimples primarily because of weight gain or the fact they haven't done any exercise since 1978.

> *Try another idea...*
> **Eating to beat cellulite is easy when you know how. Check the list of foods that help prevent it and give our dead-simple tasty recipes a try in IDEA 44, *A la carte cellulite-busting*.**

> *Here's an idea for you...*
> **OK, you may have inherited dimpled thighs from your mother, but don't let that come between you. Make it an excuse to go off and get some pampering spa or salon treatments together, when you can remind yourself of all the good things you have inherited from her.**

# Lose your inheritance

All very interesting, but what can those of us with bumpy-thighed mothers do about it? Here's your three-point strategy:

### Pick the right exercise

If your inheritance is a big bottom or wobbly thighs, you're not going to be able to turn yourself into a waif like Kate Moss. But you can create a firm, sexy rear view by adjusting your fitness routine to counteract what you've been handed down. Go for lower-body exercise that really tones and sculpts the thighs and bottom – take your pick from dancing, running, cycling or a gym routine that targets these muscle groups.

### Cut the fat

It's a simple fact that if you're genetically prone to cellulite, you won't do yourself any favours by being overweight. If you've always wanted to lose a few pounds then now, while you're in a cellulite-bashing mood, is the time to do it. Decide what your target is, based on the recommended healthy weight for your height and frame, and go for it.

If you tend to hold on to fat around your thighs and bottom, look at whether you've got too much fat in your diet. If you've got more than enough fat stored already, why load yourself up with more? Even the most heavy-bottomed of us need to consume some fat to be healthy, but a low-fat diet could be right for you. If you're a cream-in-your-coffee kind of girl, then don't try and cut out all the things you love: it'll drive you crazy and make you more likely to crack and grab something fatty. Instead, limit yourself to smaller portions of your most favourite things and take time to find tasty alternatives to the others, rather than eating something you don't enjoy.

If you don't mind a bit of calorie counting, aim for calories from fat to be no more than a third of the total for a day, then when you're comfy with that, go down to a quarter. If you're following a healthy low-fat diet, you should be getting no more than 20–25% of your calories from fat.

### Avoid oestrogen overload

There are strong indicators that the more oestrogen you have in your body, the more cellulite you're likely to get. And if you've inherited a pear shape you may also have inherited high oestrogen levels – the two often go together. There's not much you can do about that, but bear in mind that the Pill, HRT and some hormone-based treatments for acne mean you're pumping more oestrogen into your body.

## How did it go?

**Q: How come I've got cellulite but my mother hasn't?**
A: You're unlucky! It's perfectly possible to develop cellulite even if your mother's skin is still as smooth as a baby's. The gene pool is bigger than both of you.

**Q: Wasn't cellulite invented in the 1970s?**
A: The term was – but not the stuff itself. You could certainly argue that modern life contributes to cellulite – stress, processed foods, more overweight people, more sitting around on our bottoms and so on. And of course, our grandmothers weren't expected to be seen in public wearing thong bikinis, were they? But women have complained about thighs that look like cottage cheese before cottage cheese was ever heard of.

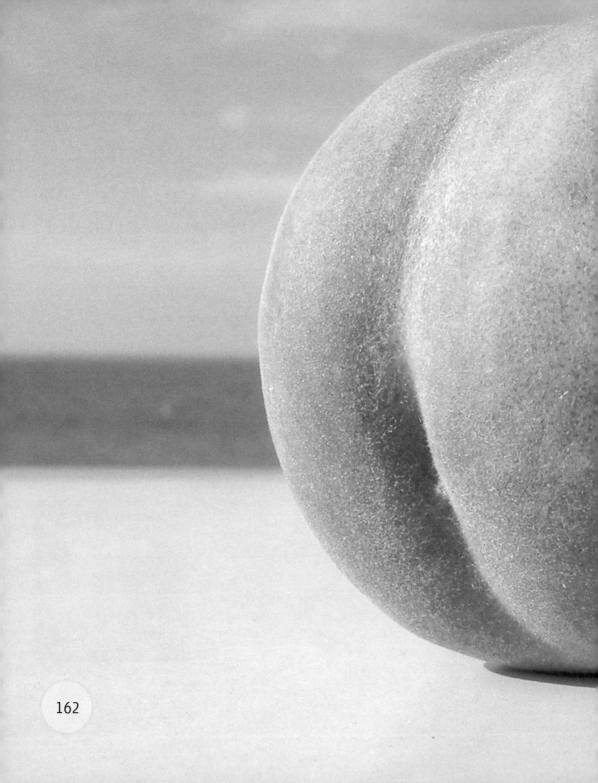

# 30

# There's a hole in my buttocks, dear Henry, dear Henry

**Why having mesotherapy injections in your bottom and thighs might not be such a bad idea. It's just a little prick...**

*A cocktail of tailor-made ingredients delivered precisely where your cellulite needs it most. Will you grin and bare it?*

That annoying saying 'You have to suffer to be beautiful' comes to mind with this treatment. Mesotherapy involves a practitioner firing a gun with a micro-fine needle at your cellulite-ridden areas,

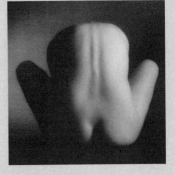

which might remind you of when you had your ears pierced. Instead of just making a hole, the needles deliver a homeopathic mix of plant extracts, drugs and vitamins into the 'mesoderm', or middle layer of the skin. The gun will be fired several times over each of your dimply patches, depending on how extensive they are.

Shooting out of these tiny needles is a mix of ingredients combined to help improve lymphatic drainage and circulation – both of which are cited regularly as vital in the battle against bulging fat cells. The cocktail of ingredients can be tailor-made to suit whoever's on the couch, which is why you need a proper consultation with the therapist first, who must be medically trained. (Remember to let the practitioner know about any health conditions you have, as this treatment doesn't suit everyone.)

The mix might include herbal extracts to boost circulation, vitamin C to help collagen production, plus any number of minerals and drugs with unpronounceable names. But the general idea is to get sluggish body systems moving to improve the look and feel of the skin.

*Here's an idea for you...*
**Want the treatments but low on cash? How about having your posterior photographed for posterity? Clinics and salons are always keen to have clients who don't mind 'before and after' pictures being taken and are willing to talk. You'll get star treatment and may be offered a discount. If not, ask for one! Go on, be cheeky and put yourself forward right now. And save some cash to spend on treatments by cutting down on booze and cigarettes – you should start seeing improvements in your cellulite as well as your bank balance.**

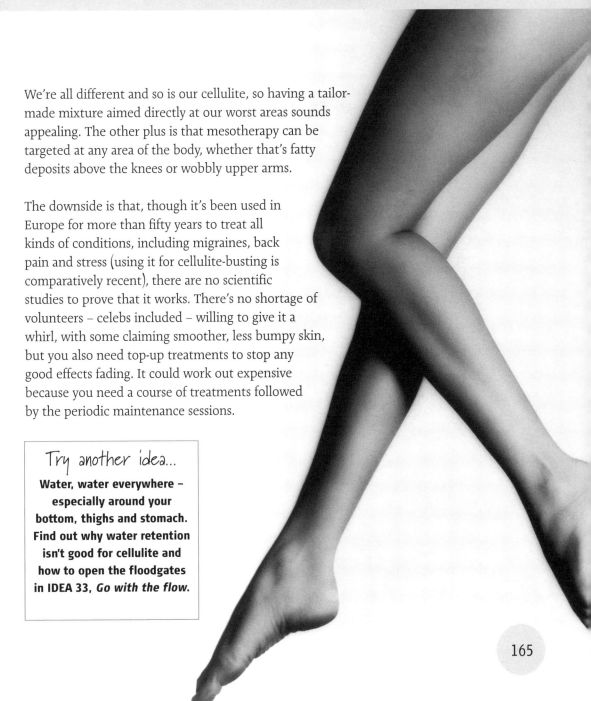

We're all different and so is our cellulite, so having a tailor-made mixture aimed directly at our worst areas sounds appealing. The other plus is that mesotherapy can be targeted at any area of the body, whether that's fatty deposits above the knees or wobbly upper arms.

The downside is that, though it's been used in Europe for more than fifty years to treat all kinds of conditions, including migraines, back pain and stress (using it for cellulite-busting is comparatively recent), there are no scientific studies to prove that it works. There's no shortage of volunteers – celebs included – willing to give it a whirl, with some claiming smoother, less bumpy skin, but you also need top-up treatments to stop any good effects fading. It could work out expensive because you need a course of treatments followed by the periodic maintenance sessions.

Try another idea...
**Water, water everywhere –
especially around your
bottom, thighs and stomach.
Find out why water retention
isn't good for cellulite and
how to open the floodgates
in IDEA 33, *Go with the flow.***

165

But back to what it feels like, so you can decide whether it's worth a shot. Pain thresholds are dramatically different among those who've braced themselves in front of the gun, some saying it's a breeze with others gritting their teeth. Don't attempt it if you have a needle phobia, but for most of the rest of us it's probably not that bad –a bit like pinpricks. The needles are normally only a few millimetres long, if that helps.

## What's the latest?

Don't fancy the needles? Happier with a bit of electric current passing through your cellulite? The next generation of mesotherapy is a version called Eporex, which uses an electrically charged roller to push the meso mixture into the skin instead of injecting it.

> ### Defining idea...
> **'There is no excellent beauty that hath not some strangeness in the proportion.'**
> FRANCIS BACON

First your thighs – or wherever the dimply bits are – are covered in the mesotherapy mixture, which includes the compound carnitine, said to help shift fat deposits. Then, while you're lying on a couch, you hold on to an electrical pad covered with conductive gel. At the same time an electrified roller is pressed up and down over your cellulite zones to push the special mesotherapy ingredients into your skin.

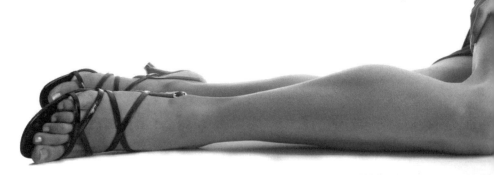

Both the rollers and the pad in your hand are wired up to the Eporex machine. There's no pain involved, say those who've had the treatment, but the hand holding the gel-covered pad jumps and jolts with the electrical current. As you're lying there on the treatment table, don't be alarmed if old black and white Frankenstein movies mysteriously come to mind.

Apparently they're hot for Eporex in Italy, where it originated, so yes, those stylish Italian women do have cellulite under their Prada. The whole thing is over in around twenty minutes. And the results? Reports are encouraging, with claims of smoother thighs and bottom after just one session, and even reduced measurements around waist and hips after several repeat treatments. Like standard mesotherapy though, you may need a series of treatments and top-up sessions.

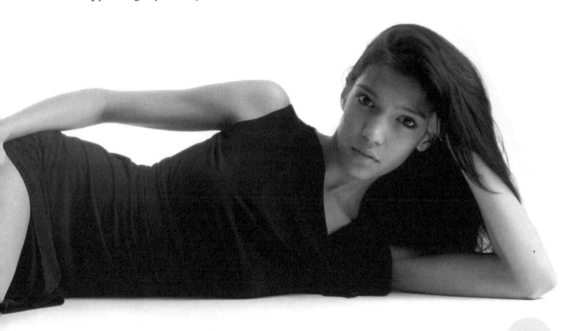

## How did it go?

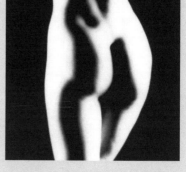

**Q: I'm slim, I do lots of exercise and eat healthily most of the time, but I've got cellulite in one place – on the sides of my legs just where they join my bottom. You can really see it in a bikini. Will mesotherapy work for me?**

A: According to practitioners, the ideal candidates for mesotherapy are those whose cellulite hasn't shifted even after diet and exercise. And because it's a localised procedure, smaller patches are easier to treat. But remember this treatment comes with no guarantees.

**Q: I still need to lose some weight but I can't stand my dimply thighs any longer. I want to have them injected right now! Do I have to wait until I'm down to my target weight?**

A: It's much better to get down to your ideal weight before you think about expensive therapies. Why spend money treating wobbly bits that might disappear anyway? If you're sticking to your exercise and healthy diet regime, you *are* doing something about your cellulite *right now*!

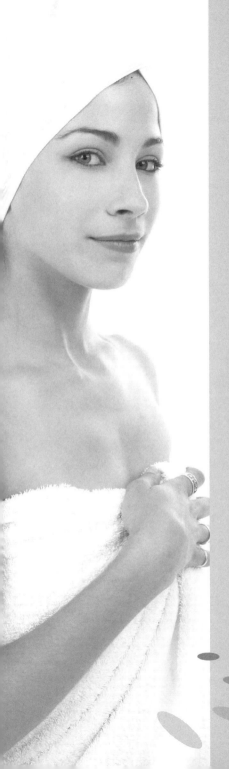

# 31

# Salon selectives

**Money no object? Mesotherapy and endermologie treatments have been combined to create a new therapy known as 'endomeso'.**

*This one involves time commitment as well as cash, but you might get quicker results.*

Want to try a salon treatment but wondering which one is best for you? Then how about a combination of two of the top therapies? There's endermologie, the deep machine massage therapy which is one of the few cellulite treatments sanctioned by the US Food and Drug Administration (FDA). And there's mesotherapy, the injection of your cellulite with a cocktail of dimple-busting ingredients.

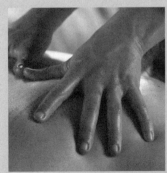

So what you'll get is a mix of deep pummelling and pulling of your flesh, plus injections in your bottom.

Sounds great, doesn't it? Well, you can't say you're not getting your money's worth. This premier league treatment is a co-ordinated big-guns attack on your cellulite. It's intensive – two salon visits a week for ten weeks. It's a bit like learning to drive by going on a two-week course instead of having a lesson a week for six months, and it means that whatever results you're going to get will be quicker.

How it works is that you have one session of endermologie on its own, then later the same week you have two back-to-back treatments: endermologie followed by mesotherapy. The idea is that the two therapies complement each other and work better together than they would on their own. The endermologie, for which the therapist uses a machine with different heads for massage and suction of the skin, is designed to pummel your cellulite into submission (bet you've felt like doing that yourself). It's meant to stretch collagen fibres and level out the bumpy look. The mesotherapy injections shoot homeopathic ingredients straight to where the cellulite is lurking, with both treatments intended to give the circulation a boost to improve skin condition.

> Here's an idea for you...
> **Fancy a few jumping jacks? Most of the expensive salon treatments for cellulite list boosting circulation as one of their benefits. But that's one thing you can do all by yourself any time – and for free. You don't even need a gym membership, and if you're stuck at home with children you can kickstart a sluggish circulation by doing jumping jacks in the garden or running on the spot. You'll notice the improvement to your skin straight away – just look at that rosy glow!**

At the same time you'll get advice on diet and exercise and other lifestyle factors affecting cellulite, and have a detailed consultation with the clinic's doctor. She will assess your health and take blood tests to check for any underlying cause that could be linked to the stubborn fat deposits.

The approach is totally focused on the individual, with the ingredients for the mesotherapy injections tailor-made to suit your very own, individual type of cellulite, with treatments fine-tuned week by week depending on how you get on.

## So, what about results?

The idea is still new, but among the relatively few women who've so far completed the course, some were impressed. But what they are impressed with seems to be more to do with inch loss than cellulite. There's nothing wrong with inch loss, if that's what you want, but it seems the cellulite is still there, if not quite so obvious. Thighs may be smoother and slightly slimmer, but this is not a case of disappearing cellulite. Maybe that would have been too much to expect, but there's also the question of how long the effects are destined to last.

Like some of the other salon cellulite treatments, any benefits have to be maintained with top-up sessions – once a month is suggested – or you could find yourself slipping back to where you started. And by the time you've had a few top-ups, it will have cost as much as liposuction, if not more.

The other snag is the time commitment: twice a week for ten weeks isn't going to be easy for a lot of us. You don't want to end up cancelling appointments at the last minute because you've gone into a frantic phase (the sort that makes you put your tights in the fridge and milk in the washing machine, which is when you really need to lie down on a salon couch). You could end up missing the benefits of regular treatment and possibly have to pay part of the cost, so checking you can commit to the full schedule is the first thing on your list.

*Try another idea...*

**If you've got a bike, you're sitting on a great way to streamline cellulitey legs and bottoms. Get pedalling and your gluteus maximus will soon be gluteus minimus. To get the most from your wheels turn to IDEA 42, *Pedal power*.**

But if you see it as an investment in yourself (and what could be better to invest in?) and it works for you, then great. You can find more details at www.cityskinklinic.co.uk.

A final thought. A big plus about salon treatments, apart from any direct improvements to your cellulite, is the benefit you get from having a 'cellulite buddy'. A bit like a training buddy, seeing your treatment therapist regularly helps keep you motivated to stick to your cellulite-shifting healthy diet, exercise regime and all the other good things you're doing to keep the crinkles at bay. Instead of expecting a specific treatment to be the Holy Grail, it's the 'whole body' approach that works best for cellulite – think holistic!

> Defining idea...
>
> **'There was a period in a woman's life when she had no cellulite, varicose veins or unsightly body hair, but she was eight at the time.'**
> KATHY LETTE, novelist

## How did it go?

**Q: Can I go straight back to work after each endomeso session?**

A: Yes. You should feel fine, though there may be bruising after the mesotherapy. Because of that, some women schedule treatment in the winter, when they're swathed in black from head to toe.

**Q: Are you sure it's safe to have all this stuff at the same time?**

A: There's been nothing to suggest it isn't, if you're healthy, but it's important to tell the doctor at the treatment centre about any health problems. You should be given a detailed questionnaire about your health before you start any treatment.

# 32

# Billy Liar?

**Your man says he doesn't know what cellulite is. Bless him. Find out what blokes really think...you may be surprised.**

Asking a man whether he can see your cellulite is a bit like saying 'Does my bum look big in this?' There's just no easy answer.

Picture the scene. There's soft music, the lights are low, there's the remains of a bottle of champagne on the table and things are hotting up for the couple on the couch.

She's the woman of his dreams and he's been gazing at her adoringly all night. Now it's getting steamy, he puts his arms around her, the satin slip she's wearing moves to reveal more of her milky-white thighs, and he whispers...'Yeeuuk, what's that dimply stuff on your legs?'

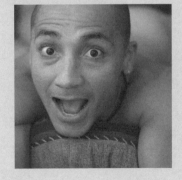

173

It doesn't happen, does it? Not in the movies, and not in real life either. No matter how much we hate our cellulitey bits, men don't seem to notice it anywhere near as much as we do. Ask yourself, have you ever been on a beach with a man who points out other women's cellulite? Thought not. He may well notice other parts of the beach babes' anatomy, but he sure as hell isn't staring at their cellulite (and let's face it, there's oceans of the stuff on beaches, whether we are talking Brighton, Bognor or Barbados). The truth is, it's women – whether they're our best friends or our biggest rivals – who notice other women's crinkly thighs, not men.

Here's an idea
for you...
If you're unlucky enough to have a man who asks you what you are going to do about your orange-peel thighs, then ditch him. Save yourself for someone who'll make you feel good about yourself, not bad.

How come? Men, it seems, see the world a little differently to women. According to academics and researchers who have studied male and female behaviour, men often look at the overall picture and skip the detail. If you have ever asked your man to pass you the butter, cheese, salami or whatever from the fridge, and wondered in amazement why he can't find it when it's staring him in the face, you'll get the idea.

But men are obsessed with women's bodies, aren't they? Well, maybe they are, but when they look at a woman they notice those well-documented signs that she's all-female: her lustrous hair, her face, her breasts, her sensuous curved shape. These are the triggers to desire that keep the human race going, and they're so powerful that the blemish on your back, the bruise on your shin or that patch of cellulite don't really get a look-in. Men are programmed to see us as attractive potential mates – objects of desire, not objects of imperfection.

Still convinced that he's lying when he says he doesn't know what you're talking about when you moan about your cellulite? Well, it may not be scientific research, but we've canvassed opinion among men of all ages, types and tastes, who have one thing in common: they're all happy to spend their lives with women who have cellulite. Here's what they say:

'I don't think she's got any cellulite.' Martin, 34

'She's always going on about her cellulite, but I can't see it.' John, 28

'I don't know what she's talking about.' Brett, 40

'She asks me if her cellulite's got any better, but I don't think she had much in the first place so I just say "Yes".' Damian, 32

'I wouldn't have noticed she had cellulite if she hadn't pointed it out to me.' Michael, 49

'I think she's got a bit of cellulite on the outside of her thighs, but it's no big deal to me.' Stuart, 50

'I quite like those dimples on her bottom.' Jim, 36

'Cell-you *what*??' Ryan, 52

Try another idea...

**When you lose weight, does it come off everywhere except where you want it to – your bottom and thighs? If the answer's yes, that could be a big clue to why you're finding it tough to smooth out those dimples. Find out more about how your body shape and hormones affect cellulite in IDEA 43,** *Ladykillers.*

Defining idea...

**'Where she's narrow, she's narrow as an arrow. And she's broad, where a broad should be broad.'**
OSCAR HAMMERSTEIN

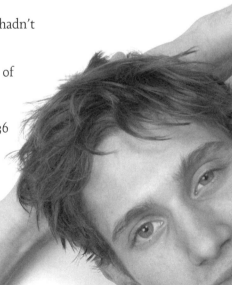

...We could go on (and on), but, you get the picture? If you want fewer dimples on your thighs to feel better, give your confidence a boost or just because you're sick of the sight of them, then fine, we are with you all the way. But if you ever start to wonder whether a man might be put off you because you've got a dimply bottom, just take another look at those quotes. So you know what to do the next time he says he can't see your cellulite, don't you? Believe him!

## How did it go?

**Q: So you mean avoiding beach holidays and taking ski trips with guys instead was a waste of time? I thought wearing a ski suit all day was the only way to stop him seeing my cellulite.**

A: Well, skiing is fun and it's great exercise for shaping your thighs. Plus it burns off so many calories you can have as many courses as you like during those long, lazy dinners in front of a log fire. And all that sun on the beach is not good for the skin, is it? So keep taking those boys to the slopes.

**Q: Before we got married my boyfriend said he couldn't see any cellulite, even though I knew it was there. Now, three years later he says he can. Did I marry the wrong man?**

A: Hold on a minute! Give the poor guy a chance. Maybe, just maybe, three years of being asked to look at your cellulite has worn him down a tiny bit and he's finally cracked. He either still can't see it and is humouring you, or because you've pointed it out so many times, he can. Either way, it doesn't mean he finds you any less desirable. The golden rule with guys, girls, is: *don't tell him it's there and he'll probably never notice it!* Remember, he's not just looking at the bits that *you* don't happen to like, but the overall, gorgeous picture.

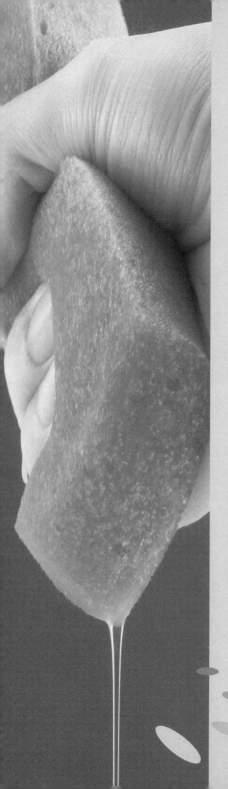

# 33

# Go with the flow

**Plagued by water retention? Discover the fluid-flushing fruit, veg and herbs that can help.**

Like cellulite itself, fluid retention is another annoying condition that seems to follow women around...but only if you let it.

You know that bloated feeling that makes your waistbands suddenly too tight and always happens just before you put on your slinkiest dress for a night out? Well if you don't, you're one of the lucky ones, but please pass this on to someone else because there are millions of women who regularly feel as if they've been blown up like a balloon.

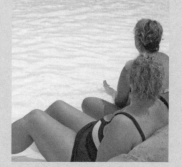

177

As you might have guessed, water retention also contributes to orange-peel skin. It has been cited over and over again by researchers investigating the causes of cellulite. The theory is that if the body holds on to too much fluid, it leaks through tiny capillary walls into the surrounding tissues and builds up in the spaces between cells, making fat cells bulge beneath the skin.

But why do we get water retention in the first place, you might ask. As far as we know, among the causes are not drinking enough water (sounds bizarre but the body tries to hang on to the fluid it's got), PMS, too much salt in the diet, and some medication and medical conditions. Sometimes persistent water retention can mean a health problem more serious than cellulite, so it's a good idea to talk to a health professional to rule this out before starting on a fluid-flushing regime.

But the good news is there are fruits, herbs and vegetables that can help, so pile your plate with these. And you know what else that means? You'll be getting your five portions of fresh fruit and veg a day. Hurrah!

Here's an idea
for you...
You can grow parsley easily on your kitchen windowsill so you've always got a handy supply of this fluid-flushing herb. Throw it in soups, sprinkle it on fish dishes, omelettes, on salads and in sandwiches. When you get it as a garnish in restaurants, don't leave it on the side of your plate – eat it!

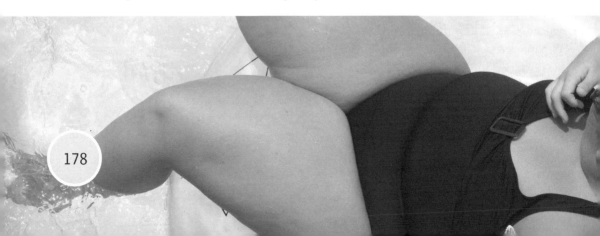

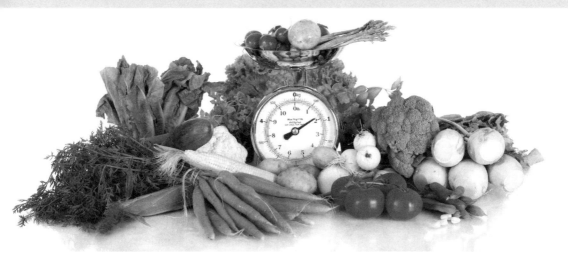

# Veg it out

Try upping your intake of some of these to encourage your body to flush out excess fluid.

**Asparagus** is a natural diuretic and contains potassium, one of the minerals that helps prevent water retention. A spring vegetable, it's widely available and best value fresh in May, so make the most of it then. You can still buy it out of season in the smarter supermarkets. Just simmer asparagus tips for about 5–8 minutes depending on thickness (steaming is even better), add butter and serve.

**Avocados** are potassium-rich and stuffed with vitamin E, which is good for the skin. For a quick snack just halve, scoop out the stone and shake some of your favourite salad dressing into the dip.

**Spinach** and other green leafy vegetables are loaded with magnesium, which helps keep the correct balance of the body's fluids. Spinach goes well with eggy things (omelettes, poached eggs, eggs florentine), but cook it very lightly to avoid it going soggy. Don't forget raw spinach in supermarket salad bags too.

*Try another idea...*

**Give your skin a chance to stop the cellulite bulging through by making sure it's in peak condition. Turn to IDEA 22, *Getting a skinful*, for the foods with the skin-boosting nutrients.**

179

**Cucumber** is a mild diuretic. Always have one in the fridge and slice it into sandwiches, chop it into salads, and use as a dipper with hummous or sour cream and chives.

**Celery** is another watery vegetable that's a natural diuretic. Use as a crudité with a dip before dinner, and keep some washed and ready as a snack any time. But try not to dip it in salt please.

**Broccoli** is one of the 'superfoods' that is so packed with nutrients it multi-tasks all over the body. Contains fluid-busting potassium. Steam or simmer for five minutes only so as not to lose any of those vital vitamins, or better still wash and eat raw dipped in hummous. Delicious.

Salty foods, of course, are a no-no if you're prone to fluid retention, and if you're still in the habit of throwing a pinch or two of salt into the pan when you're cooking vegetables, then hide the salt at the back of the cupboard. Our parents and grandparents used to salt anything that was green, to 'bring out the flavour', but chances are you'll never notice the difference.
If you do, sprinkle herbs in the cooking water instead.

The same goes for the habit of sprinkling salt on food at the table. You just don't need it, and if you don't put any salt on the table in the first place you'll soon forget about it. Cruets are *sooo* last century.

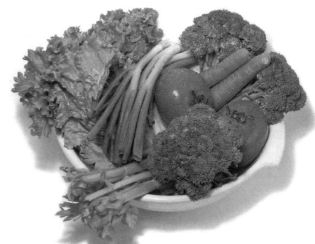

180

## Fruit to go

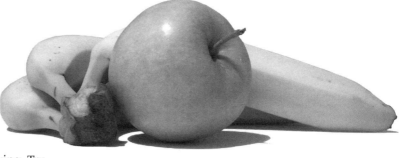

**Apples** are a good source of fluid-flushing potassium and the fibre pectin, which helps keep your system moving. Try good old-fashioned baked apples like your granny used to make.

**Oranges** contain potassium and fibre and so many vitamins you should eat one every day.

**Bananas** are another potassium-rich fruit. You can't get enough of 'em, so chop on cereals or have as a mid-morning or afternoon snack. We know women who are never without a banana in their handbags.

**Kiwi fruit**, another diuretic, is great with Greek yoghurt, or throw in the juicer with banana and other fruits if you find the flavour too sharp.

**Grapefruit** is good for fibre and potassium and is often used as a detoxifier. Go for the sweeter pink ones if you're not keen on the acidic taste.

## Herbs and teas

**Fennel** This aniseed-scented herb is known as a powerful diuretic. Drink as a herbal tea, or you can mix fennel essential oil into body cream and massage into your thighs. Follow advice about the amount of drops to use carefully when using essential oils as they can be very powerful (don't use if pregnant or epileptic).

**Parsley** A particularly good diuretic. Contains a chemical called coumarin which helps diminish water retention.

**Camomile** A calming herb that is used for both PMS and water retention. Sip camomile tea whenever you feel bloated.

**Nettle** Highly recommended by herbalists to combat fluid retention. Drink as a tea (it is an acquired taste, but worth acquiring).

**Dandelion** (What is it with weeds?) Stimulates urine flow, so drink the herbal tea or harvest leaves from your own back garden, wash thoroughly and add to your salad bowl.

## How did it go?

**Q: Someone told me drinking cider vinegar was a cure for water retention. Doesn't it taste terrible though?**
A: You don't have to drink it neat! Add it to a small cup of hot water and knock it back like medicine, then take a big bite of an apple.

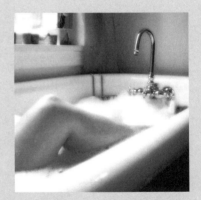

**Q: Why don't men get water retention?**
A: They do, but not as much as women. Basically, it's your hormones, dear. Fluctuations in hormone levels during the menstrual cycle and around the time of the menopause are believed to be among the causes, plus some women on the Pill tend to get more water retention. Sometimes it's hard to be a woman...

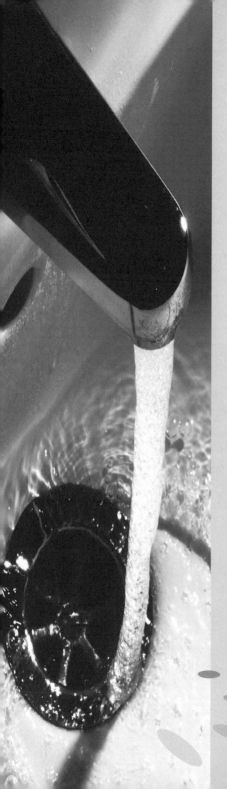

# 34

# Softly, softly

**Manual lymphatic drainage sounds like a serious plumbing problem, but is in fact an effective, gentle touch massage that's so delicate you wouldn't believe it could work.**

It's one of the best kept secrets in the beauty business and it can only be performed by highly trained practitioners. But MLD is described as the best massage treatment there is for cellulite — so lie down and enjoy!

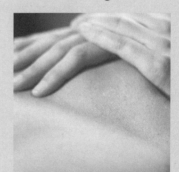

You are going to love this one. MLD is a type of massage like no other – it feels like you're being stroked with a feather by a fairy. It's not the kind of massage that gets knots out of tense muscles or boosts blood flow, but instead uses gentle, rhythmic movements to stimulate the body's lymphatic system.

Here's an idea
for you...
If you're pregnant and feeling like a stranded whale, book yourself some MLD sessions because it helps reduce swollen legs and ankles. And – joy of joys – it can reduce stretchmarks too.

## What's the lymphatic system?

The lymphatic system is a vast network of tiny tubes which carry lymph, a colourless fluid, around the body. The lymphatic system operates like a drainage unit, with the lymph carrying waste products and harmful substances out of the body. It all sounds very efficient and it is, as long as it works properly. In a way it is similar to the blood circulation system. But while the circulatory system has a pump, the heart, the lymphatic system doesn't and can become slow and sluggish and less able to rid the body of toxins and excess fluid, which contributes to the formation of cellulite.

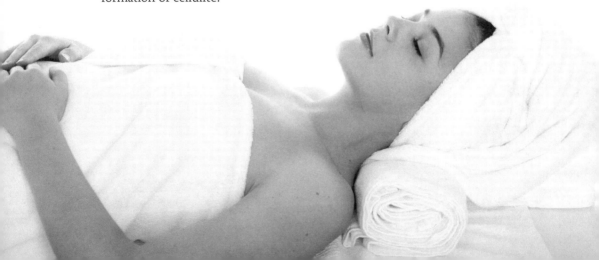

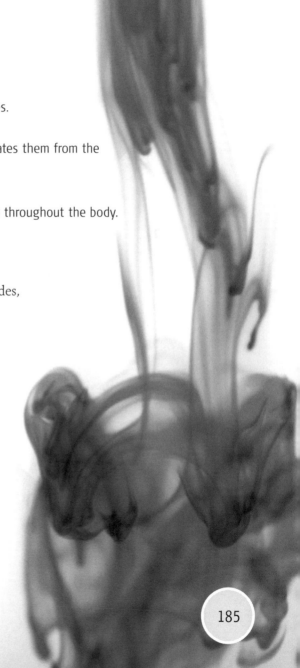

# What does the lymph do?

- It gets rid of excess fluid from the body tissues.

- It breaks down harmful substances and eliminates them from the body - viruses, bacteria, waste products.

- It transports vitamins, nutrients and hormones throughout the body.

- It strengthens the body's immune system.

The waste products are carried to the lymph nodes, which are like cleansing stations, located in the neck, armpits, abdomen and groin. The harmful substances are processed in the nodes before entering the bloodstream and being carried on to the liver for detoxification and excretion.

You know when you have a cold and the glands in your neck get a bit swollen and sometimes sore? Those are the lymph nodes, doing their job of trying to get all the toxic stuff out of your body.

## How does it work on cellulite?

MLD is primarily linked to the reduction of cellulite through the elimination of excess fluid (or water retention), and most therapists agree that water retention is nearly always present in cellulite sufferers.

Other ways MLD could help cellulite, although not proven, are through the removal of toxins, and the breaking up of fat cells – the lymph is capable of transporting fat cells. If you accept the idea that cellulite is partly caused by the build-up of toxins, then it makes sense that the lymphatic system, which helps remove waste products from the body, could play an important role in reducing it.

*Try another idea...*

**Love to slather butter on your toast, pour cream on your puddings and mix mayonnaise with your tuna? Too many fatty foods are doing your cellulite no favours whatsoever. For ways to swap them for equally tasty alternatives go straight to IDEA 11, *Goodbye Mr Chips.***

## What happens during a session?

The therapist uses gentle rhythmic pumping movements to move the skin in the direction of the lymph flow, so that the lymph moves more freely towards the nodes. Treatment always includes the neck, because lymph nodes are located there, and for cellulite the buttocks, thighs and abdomen will also be targeted. Although it's very gentle, it's also a deeply relaxing therapy.

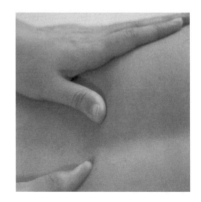

# Health benefits

There's not much doubt that MLD can do great
things for the body – its medical benefits are
proven and used all over the world. One of its
major uses is to help people recover after surgery
by reducing post-op swelling (lymphoedema),

Defining idea...
**'Why do we pay for
psychotherapy when
massages cost half as
much?'**
JASON LOVE

caused by the build-up of lymphatic fluid. MLD is also used to improve sinusitis,
rheumatoid arthritis, acne and other skin problems, as well as boosting healing after
injuries such as fractures, sprains and burns.

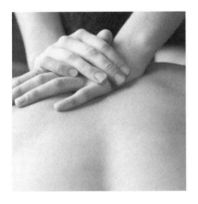

The lymph system is linked with fighting disease
so stimulation with massage might help the body
to heal itself of all kinds of problems. Tell your
therapist about any health concerns before your
treatment and she may be able to adapt the
massage to benefit more than your cellulite.

## How to find a therapist

MLD sessions will probably cost slightly more
than other forms of massage because of the highly specialised nature of the training
involved. As with other forms of treatment, you should always check the credentials
of a therapist before you book any sessions. MLD practitioners have their own
professional bodies (in the UK check out the website of the Association of Manual
Lymphatic Drainage Practitioners: www.mlduk.org.uk). Therapists have to be
trained using one of several internationally recognised training methods, and have
to keep up to date with MLD developments by attending review classes a minimum
of once every two years.

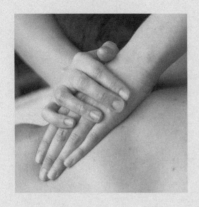

## How did it go?

**Q: How many MLD sessions will I have to have before I notice a difference in my cellulite?**

A: This is definitely not a one-off treatment and you will usually need around ten sessions before you notice any difference. How much and how quickly MLD improves your cellulite varies according to how severe it is and how long you have had it. However, therapists say that all cases of cellulite can be improved, and clients will always notice a difference, particularly if they are following a whole-lifestyle approach to reduce it, including good diet and exercise.

**Q: I have heard that dry skin brushing helps lymphatic drainage. Is this true?**

A: Yes. Although it doesn't specifically target lymph drainage in the way that MLD does, dry skin brushing can help boost the lymphatic system and is a good supplementary treatment. You will need to do it very regularly to get the benefits, once a day or twice if possible. Just get into the habit of putting your toothbrush down and picking up your body brush!

## 35

# Up in arms

**The rebellion against crinkly upper arms starts here. Yes, you *can* wear sleeveless dresses again.**

As if cellulite on the nether regions wasn't enough, some of us have got it on the backs of our arms too. But it doesn't have to stay there, there's a lot you can do to shift it — without even leaving your sofa.

A much smaller percentage of women have cellulite on their upper arms compared to those who get it on their thighs and bottoms, but for those who do it's just as annoying and confidence-denting as getting it anywhere else – if not more so. Your arms are so much more visible, and most people cursed with crepey skin here would give their right arm (well that's one way of getting shot of it) to be cellulite-free. Who wants to wear long sleeves all summer and never get to slink around in a strappy evening dress?

Just like the hips and bottom, women are genetically predisposed to store fat on their upper arms. Fat accumulation here also tends to get worse the older we get. You've heard the one about women over forty being advised not to wave anyone goodbye while wearing a sleeveless dress? Batwings, bingo wings or whatever other unflattering name you want to give them, it's this wobbly excess flesh that attracts cellulite like wasps to a jar of jam.

> Here's an idea
> for you...
> **Look for dresses with wispy chiffon sleeves – the sheer fabric will give your arms just enough camouflage but will still look glamorous and sexy.**

It's possible to be quite slim and still have wobbly upper arms, so it's not only those who are carrying excess weight that are vulnerable – but the first thing to do to get rid of cellulite here is to shed the pounds if you're over your ideal weight. If you're prone to cellulite in this area you can't afford to carry excess baggage.

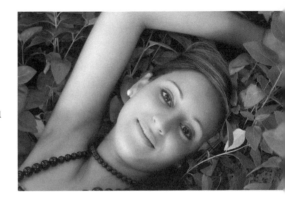

## Not waving but toning

The next thing to do is to really tone up your upper arms – it can take years off your overall appearance. Madonna and Jerry Hall have reached the flabby arm age but you don't see them waving batwings at their fans. If they can do it, so can you. You don't need a personal trainer or any expensive equipment either.

Think about the general exercise you're doing at the moment – how much of it involves your upper arms? Maybe you're running and cycling, but you're not doing much for your upper body. Try swimming – both front crawl and breaststroke will help you trim down and sculpt upper arms. Both use powerful tricep movements, and pushing against the water adds resistance.

> *Try another idea...*
> **Give your arm cellulite a thorough pummelling with endermologie, a deep massage treatment. Find out more by turning to IDEA 6,** *Can you feel the force?*

If you're a walker, don't just shove your hands in your pockets, buy a couple of Nordic walking poles (available from sports shops) and give your arms a workout as well as your legs. Nordic walking, during which you swing your poles rhythmically to help you along, really uses the muscles on the backs of the arms *and* burns extra calories.

# Best home exercise: tricep dips

The tricep dip is a simple exercise to tone up flabby skin on the underside of the arms and help diminish cellulite.

■ Sit on a dining chair, bench or even the side of the bath, gripping the edge of the seat/bath or placing your palms flat down on the surface, close to your body.

■ Put your legs out in front with your feet flat on the floor – the further away your feet are the more you will work your triceps.

■ Using your arms to support yourself, ease your body forwards and drop your bottom almost to the floor, then return to your starting position.

■ Repeat 10–20 times, rest and then do another set. Do as many sets as you can – at least three or four – and nearly every day of the week if possible. It only takes a matter of minutes and the more you do the quicker the results.

## Roll your sleeves up

You may be able to improve the look of the back of cellulitey arms by self-massage. As it's a small area it doesn't take long and you don't have to take your clothes off, so you could do it any time you've got a spare few minutes. Buy some massage oil or rich body lotion and use firm, circular movements and some gentle kneading.

## Is cosmetic surgery an option?

Yes, but it's a drastic measure and will leave scars on the underside of your upper arms, sometimes reaching as far down as the elbow. It's sometimes considered for those who have lost a lot of weight quickly and are left with loose skin that no amount of arm exercises seems to shift completely.

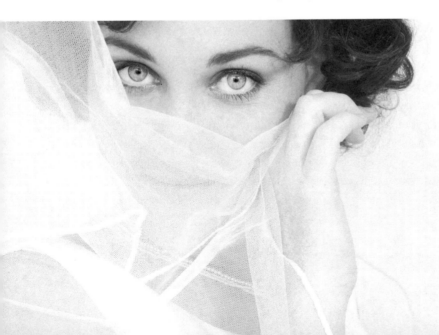

193

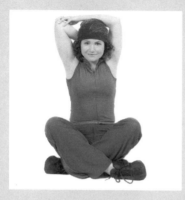

How did it go?

**Q: Does dry skin brushing help cellulite on the arms like it does on the thighs?**

A: Yes, and, as you would on your lower body, you should brush in the direction of the heart to stimulate lymphatic drainage – so brush from the elbow to the armpit.

**Q: I don't have cellulite on the back of my arms but I've got lots of tiny bumps like minute pimples – they make my arms feel really rough. Are they the beginnings of cellulite? And how can I get rid of them?**

A: This is not the beginnings of cellulite, it's a common complaint and is likely to be caused by the skin becoming slightly dry, particularly in winter when we spend most of our time in centrally heated environments. Give the area a good exfoliation with a body scrub every time you're in the bath or shower to encourage cell turnover, then afterwards massage with a heavy moisturiser, such as those formulated for dry skin.

**Q: I hardly have time for exercise. Have you got any tips on how I can fit this in to my busy day?**

A: Who cleans your windows? Think twice before you pay a window cleaner. It's great exercise for the upper arms, so get the Windolene out and save yourself some money. If you do it once a week you'll get a good workout and have the cleanest windows in the street. Or keep a set of hand weights next to the sofa. Every time you sit down to watch the news or your favourite soap, use them to trim your triceps.

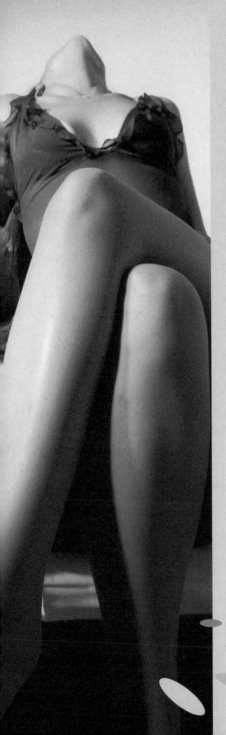

# 36

# The lady vanishes

**Look inches slimmer with figure-flattering hosiery made from skin-massaging materials – anti-cellulite tights. We kid you not.**

*Don't want to wear short skirts? Worried about lumps and bumps showing through slinky clothes? Try these on for thighs...*

Of all the 'cellulite-busting' cures out there, this sounds one of the weirdest. Anything you can do without any effort – though it's a bit of an effort pulling some of these tights on – is always going to be tempting. There are several versions of anti-cellulite hosiery, which claim to work in different ways, from micro-massaging the legs to delivering sea minerals to the thighs.

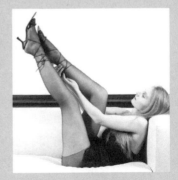

# Tights with caffeine

As drinking too much caffeine has been linked to restricting blood flow and circulation – which is bad for your cellulite – it might seem odd to be slapping it on your skin. However, it is known through laboratory experiments that caffeine can boost the metabolism of cells it penetrates, and it can also be absorbed through the skin.

So impregnating tights with caffeine may not be as crazy as it sounds. Microscopic gelatine capsules containing caffeine are woven into the tights. Your body heat breaks down the capsules, allowing the caffeine to be absorbed through the skin. The idea is that the caffeine increases the metabolism and burns fat if the tights are worn every day for between one and four weeks, resulting in losing centimetres from thighs and diminishing the orange-peel effect.

*Here's an idea for you...*

When you want to wear short skirts that show your thighs and backs of your legs in summer, those all-concealing opaque black numbers don't look quite right. Instead choose high-denier, light-coloured ones with plenty of Lycra, which will hold you firmly enough to smooth out the dimples.

When they were first launched, the tights sold out in Europe within ten days of hitting the shops. They look like normal tights, they're 20 denier and come in skin tone or black. Dieticians have questioned whether there is enough caffeine in the tights to have a genuine effect. However, some wearers who measured their thighs before and after three weeks of wearing the tights reported losing several centimetres. If you want to give them a try you can buy them on www.palmersshop.com or www.tightsplease.co.uk. They cost about three times more than standard good-quality tights and the caffeine will last for five washes before it becomes ineffectual.

# Cellulite-massaging tights

There are several versions of tights on the market that claim to be made of a 'microweave' that massages the skin as you move around, stimulating the skin's microcirculation, easing water retention and reducing cellulite.

**Try another idea...**
What can cellulite creams really do for you? Are the most expensive ones that different from the rest? Find out by turning to IDEA 8, *On the shelf.*

There seems to be no independent scientific proof to back up this theory, but, as with the caffeine tights, some wearers who tested them reported improvements, including less obvious orange-peel skin and reduced thigh circumference after several weeks' wear, as well as firmer and smoother skin. Some people also said they could feel the massaging effect as they walked around.

Versions of these tights come in different deniers and some have control tops, but they all tend to be more expensive than the caffeine version. Check out what's available at www.indigohealth.co.uk or www.pantyhose-stockings-hosiery.com.

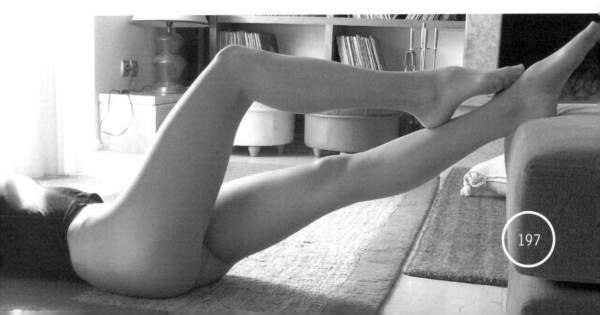

# Give yourself a 'leg lift'

Other versions of anti-cellulite tights follow the 'compression' technique, starting with a very tight fit at the ankles which gradually lessens as you move up the leg. These 'compression' tights are very similar to support tights, which are worn for medical reasons and designed to prevent varicose veins by boosting circulation.

The graduated compression means the blood circulation is encouraged up the legs and back towards the heart, giving the venous system a boost – and better circulation is supposed to be good for cellulite. So could wearing a pair of your granny's support tights have a positive effect on cellulite?

Scholl – one of the major manufacturers of support hosiery – makes no claims that any of its products can diminish the dimpley stuff. But they do say that support tights could have a 'cosmetic' effect on cellulite-ridden legs. Support tights provide a gravity-defying 'leg lift' which gives everything a better shape – calves, fat above the knees and thighs.

# Body-contouring tights

The secret weapons in countless women's underwear drawers are tights with hold-you-in control pants. They don't claim to make any difference to cellulite, except for squashing it flat so lumps and bumps cannot be detected.

These are the tights to go for if you are unlucky enough to have cellulite that can be seen through thin, close-fitting fabrics, such as silky evening skirts or trousers. Tights under trousers might seem a no-no, but they also have the great advantage of avoiding the VPL.

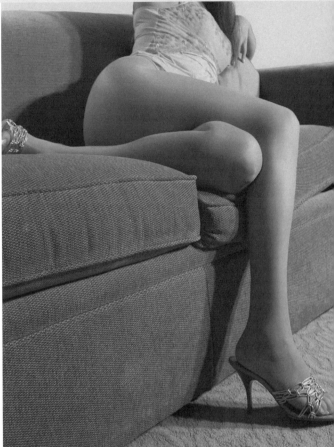

If you want to smooth out 'saddle-bag' thighs as well, the tights where the reinforced section comes down the thighs a few inches do a great job.

**Tip 1** Don't try and wear underwear with these control-top tights – there's no need and if you do the panels are so tight when you pull them on that they will make your knickers roll up, causing ridges underneath the tights.

**Tip 2** Be careful if you like to wear short skirts – some of the control-top tights that come halfway down the thighs like cycling shorts could be dodgy, particularly when you're climbing stairs. Control tops visible under your mini might not be a good look.

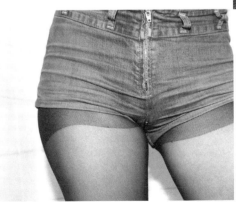

Avoid shiny tights. Whether black or neutral, anything that reflects light will make your legs look bigger and draw attention to them – not ideal if you've got something you want to hide.

199

## How did it go?

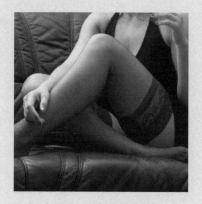

### Q: Can I wear these control tights all the time?

A: Yes, there's no reason why you can't – in fact if they're going to have any effect you should wear them on a daily basis. Medical compression hosiery, which is worn to help blood circulation, is normally worn daily. Remember to take the tights off before you go to bed though!

### Q: I've read about tights impregnated with sea minerals that can improve cellulite. Are these any good?

A: Dermatologists say there is insufficient evidence to suggest that hosiery containing minerals extracted from marine plants – which are used in thalassotherapy to treat cellulite – could have much of an effect. What they may do, though, is moisturise your legs and make them feel smoother and sexier.

> Defining idea...
> *'It seems to me we can never give up longing and wishing while we are thoroughly alive.'*
> GEORGE ELIOT

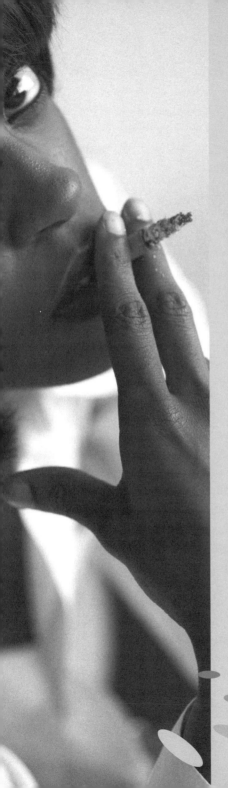

# 37

# Smoke gets in your eyes (and bottom and thighs)

**Cigarettes make cellulite worse. Another good reason to 'just say no'.**

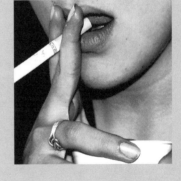

If you're almost ready to give up smoking but need one more incentive to drop that pack of twenty in the bin, just think that some of the great things you're doing to reduce your cellulite will be wiped out the next time you light up.

201

A build up of toxins in your body and poor circulation are two of the things that can lead to cellulite. So what does smoking do to your body (apart from increase your risk of cancers, clog up your arteries and bring on an early menopause)? You guessed it – it slows down your circulation and prevents toxins from being eliminated from your system efficiently.

You only have to look at the skin of someone who's smoked all their life to know that smoking and glowing, healthy skin don't exactly go together. Cigarettes reduce blood and oxygen flow to the skin and send those dodgy free radicals to weaken the collagen – just when collagen is what you need to keep the dimple-making fat cells under control.

So get whatever help you can to give up – check out the how-to-quit websites, helplines and support groups. Nicotine replacement therapy – skin patches, chewing gum, tablets and even nasal sprays – has been shown to double your chances of giving up successfully compared to relying solely on willpower.

'Stop smoking' clinics have also proved a hit: those who make it through the doors are up to four times more likely to manage to ditch the weed than those who go it alone.

With hypnosis and acupuncture, you pay your money and take your chance. There is less evidence to show that they work as consistently as nicotine replacement, but they make all the difference to some people, so don't hold back if you think that could be the answer for you.

There are some amazing sounding drugs being developed to help desperate smokers, such as one to prevent the brain allowing you to feel satisfaction from smoking, but don't hold your breath – these are a few years down the line.

## A little extra help

- If you can't face going cold turkey, postpone the time you light a cigarette by an hour every day. By the time you get to midnight, you know you've won!

- Keep some of your old stale butts in an ashtray and sniff them every time you're tempted. They'll smell worse by the day.

- If a cigarette at the end of a meal is one of your 'triggers', do something else, like going and brushing your teeth. Not as much fun, but it helps!

- Plan a treat for the end of every week you get through without smoking.

- When you're tempted, ring someone you know who's given up for support and tips.

Here's an idea
for you...
**Ask ten of the friends who keep nagging you to give up smoking to put their money where their mouths are. Get them to bet you £10 that you can't go a month without a cigarette. Think of the agony of having to shell out £100 if you fail, and if you win (of course you will!) use the money to treat yourself to some pampering anti-cellulite treatments. And if you've gone a month without lighting up, you know you can crack it for good...**

# Ten other good reasons to give up smoking

**Try another idea...**

It's not only thighs and bottoms that are susceptible to cellulite. If you've noticed it creeping along your upper arms, you're not alone. Turn to IDEA 35, *Up in arms*, for some easy ways to wave it goodbye.

1.  All that lip pursing action when you suck up the nicotine gives you vertical lines around your lips. You've seen those old ladies with lipstick bleeding into the creases around their mouths, haven't you? That's you, baby.

2.  It dries up the skin on your face too, giving you premature wrinkles.

3.  It decreases your fertility. And if you do have children, remember: your smoke is seriously bad for their health.

4.  Think of the money. Every year the price of cigarettes goes up and your bank balance goes down. And with the cash you save you could afford a whole series of pampering anti-cellulite treatments.

5.  Smoking diminishes the beneficial effects of vitamin C, one of the most powerful and important vitamins your body needs.

6. With the number of places you can't smoke increasing faster than you can say 'dimples', your social life is going to take a hammering. Soon you'll be asking for a table for one down at the Fag End and Firkin.

7. Improve your job prospects. Ticking the 'smoker' box on your dream job application form puts you in the 'no' pile pronto.

8. Get more boyfriends. Dating agencies say that no matter how attractive, stylish or sparkling a woman's personality, only a very small percentage of men are willing to go out with a girl who keeps a packet of Marlboros in her Prada bag.

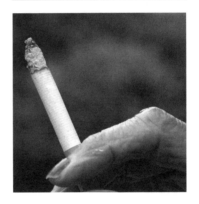

9. Food tastes better. Chemicals and tar from cigarettes coat the inside of a smoker's mouth, including the taste buds.

10. You'll be able to smile again. Tar discolours your teeth, and there are few things more unattractive and ageing than stained teeth.

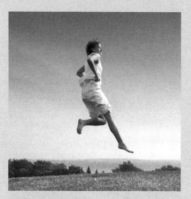

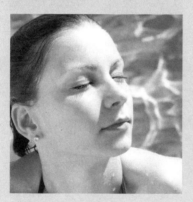

# How did it go?

**Q: How long after I give up smoking will I notice the effect on my cellulite?**

A: When you stop smoking your body begins to repair the damage caused by cigarettes almost immediately. How long before you notice a difference will depend on what other factors are affecting your cellulite, but the improvements to circulation, which will help the condition of the skin including the places you have cellulite, can start about two weeks after giving up. The toxins nicotine and carbon monoxide will be eliminated from the body after 48 hours.

**Q: Will I put on weight when I give up smoking?**

A: Not if you are eating healthily and getting enough exercise. Giving up smoking is the perfect time to take up some exercise you'll enjoy, such as dancing or cycling. If you're going to substitute smoking with snacking, then your weight will go up. Just be aware of the times when you most want a cigarette and make sure you're doing something you enjoy to distract you.

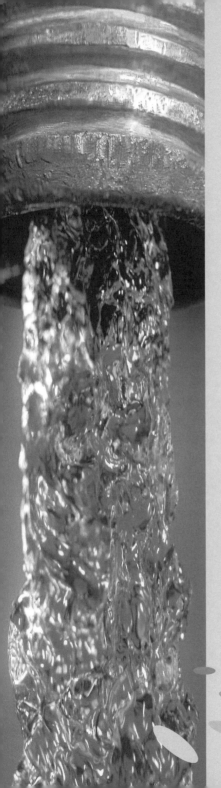

# 38

# Suck it and see

**Liposuction. It's surgery, it's drastic, but it does what it says on the tin: it sucks the fat out of your bottom and thighs.**

We've all dreamed of waking up one day to find that all the crinkly, lumpy bits have disappeared overnight. Abracadabra: no cellulite.

It's the instantaneousness of liposuction that tempts us. No more staring in the mirror week after week to see if there's any improvement, no more ten-week regimes – just whoosh! and it's gone. So is liposuction really the answer for cellulite?

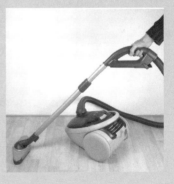

One thing's for sure: you'll certainly notice a difference after liposuction. Surgeons have removed as much as three litres of fat in one session, resulting in the bottom or thighs measuring quite a few centimetres less.

But it's expensive, not without risk and discomfort, and does not remove all your cellulite – since it doesn't tackle the cause of it. Because it sucks fat out of your body and some of that fat is cellulite, you will have less cellulite. So in a way it's simply a drastic and instant form of weight loss – you might go from having a size 12 bottom with cellulite to having a size 10 bottom with cellulite.

> Here's an idea for you...
>
> **If you're considering liposuction, get down to your ideal weight first. As cellulite is a form of fat, if you lose excess weight some of your cellulite will go with it. Once you've got down to your 'fighting weight' you can reassess your cellulite to see if you can deal with the remaining dimples with a less drastic form of treatment.**

## So who does it work for?

Women who are very pear-shaped, so that their bottom half is out of proportion to the top half, are most likely to benefit from liposuction to improve their cellulite. That's those of us who, if we're brave enough to buy a bikini, are tempted to swap the bottom part for one two sizes bigger.

For these unlucky ladies, no matter how much they diet and exercise, the bottom-heavy shape will still remain. Their bodies are simply genetically predisposed to hang on to fat cells below the waist, like a terrier hanging on to a bone when all the other dogs have let go. This may have been nature's way of ensuring females had enough fat cells to support a pregnancy in times of famine, but the knowledge that you could live off your fat longer than anyone else if you're lost in the Peruvian jungle is little consolation when all you want to do is look reasonable on the beach.

Women with this shape have been known to end up with hollow cheekbones and a boney chest while their bottoms – though reduced from dieting and toned from exercise – would still make J-Lo proud. And, if they are also genetically cellulite-prone, possibly because they have high levels of oestrogen, those bottoms will still be dimply.

If they can't just glory in being a J-Lo shape and accept that cellulite goes with the territory, then liposuction can at least reduce the size of their bottom half and give their figures more of a balanced hour-glass shape.

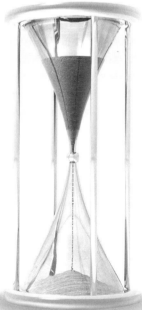

In reducing the amount of fat, liposuction will reduce the amount of cellulite, simply because you're going to end up with a smaller bottom and/or slimmer thighs. But some cellulite will still remain, and if you put on weight it is likely to increase again. However, being more in proportion may be worth it. Hour-glass or pear? Only you can decide.

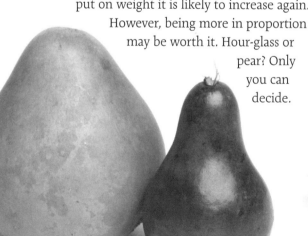

Try another idea...

**More muscle means less fat – and less cellulite. Getting a more muscular body doesn't mean looking like a wrestler – think Madonna, not Schwarzenegger. Find out how to develop muscle and lose cellulite by turning to IDEA 10, *I want muscles.***

## What actually happens?

Liposuction is usually performed under a general anaesthetic. Several small incisions are made to allow a narrow cannula or tube to access the fat underneath the skin. The fat is then suctioned out through the tube.

## The risks

You'll run the same risks with liposuction that you get with any surgery, including infection, bleeding or fluid overload from the anaesthetic. With liposuction, if too much fat and fluid is removed the body can go into shock and the blood pressure drop drastically, which could be fatal. So doing your research and making sure you only put your bottom in the hands of an experienced surgeon with an established track record goes without saying.

## Swelling and scarring

The instant results actually take a few weeks to become clear. Post-operative puffiness and swelling mean that you don't get to see the full benefits of the surgeon's handiwork until your body's had a chance to recover. The holes where the cannulas have been inserted will leave scars, but these should be small and hopefully in places where few people get the chance to see them. Obviously you're not going to get away with having all this done without it hurting, but, like most surgery, discomfort can be controlled with painkillers.

# Will my cellulite come back?

Yes, definitely if you put on weight, and probably if you stop exercising or your healthy diet goes out of the window. The surgery will have removed some of the cellulite but it will have done nothing to prevent the underlying cause of the stuff – whether that's genetic or hormonal, exacerbated by junk food, a couch-potato lifestyle or whatever. So the message is clear – if you're going to go to the trouble and expense of liposuction, there's even more reason to eat well, exercise and do all the other things that keep cellulite at bay, not less. There's no escape!

> Defining idea...
> **'I'm tired of all this nonsense about beauty being only skin-deep. That's deep enough. What do you want – an adorable pancreas?'**
> JEAN KERR

# How did it go?

**Q: Would liposuction be a good idea to get rid of the cellulite over my knees?**
A: Liposuction can work reasonably well for fatty deposits over the knees because it is quite a small area. It's also an area that you cannot make much difference to with diet and exercise.

**Q: I've heard that liposuction doesn't work if you're over a certain age. Is it true?**
A: Some surgeons are cautious about offering liposuction to older women, such as anyone over fifty, because the skin is not as elastic as that of younger women so could sag once fat has been removed. The excess skin can be removed, as it would be with a 'tummy tuck', but that would entail another surgical procedure.

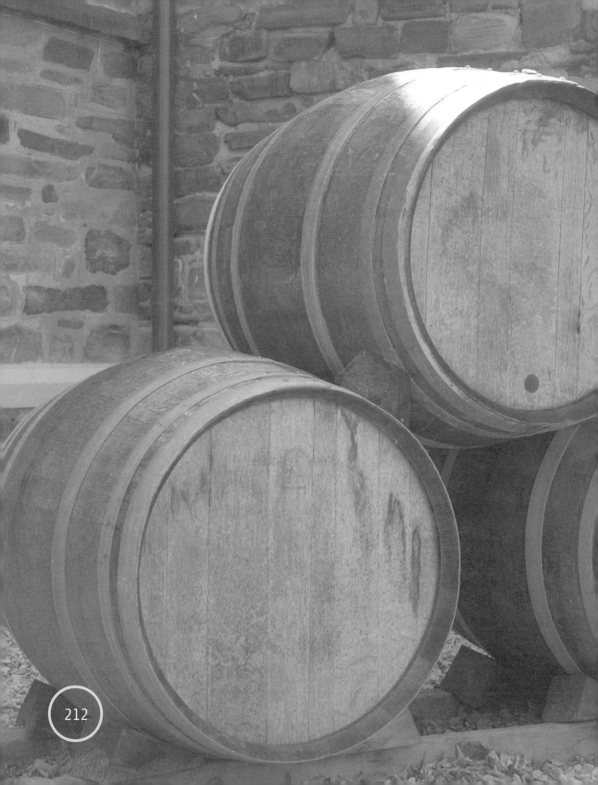

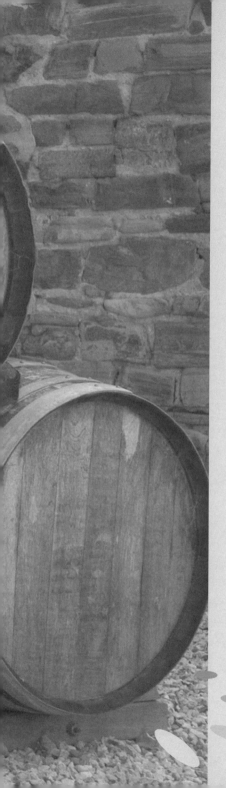

# 39

# Scraping the barrel

**A blast of fine crystals can exfoliate the top layer of skin and reduce the puckering effect. Large, wobbly behinds can really benefit from this microdermabrasion treatment.**

*If microdermabrasion can reduce fine lines and wrinkles on the face, think what it could do for your bottom!*

Don't like the look of the skin on your bottom? Then scrape it off! Microdermabrasion, a favourite treatment with celebrities, is used regularly in salons and spas to soften the appearance of facial creases and wrinkles by scouring off the surface skin. If you're squeamish you may feel you've read enough already – but there is no shortage of devotees

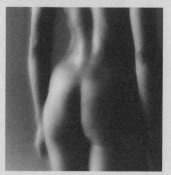

who keep coming back for more. Some of these use microdermabrasion to help with acne, birthmarks or scars, but for most it's an anti-ageing treatment that leaves the skin silky soft and with a healthy looking glow.

But the skin on the body can benefit too – microdermabrasion is often recommended for spotty backs and stretch marks. So what about the regions where cellulite roams free – the bottom, thighs and backs of the legs? The truth is that microdermabrasion cannot make cellulite disappear, but it can make the skin in these areas – which are also prone to developing rough, dry patches and tiny spots – look and feel a lot smoother and healthier. And it's said that the treatment can stimulate the production of collagen, which helps prevent cellulite by keeping the fat underneath the skin in place.

> *Here's an idea for you...*
>
> **A good exfoliation of the cellulite-prone areas of your bottom, thighs or upper arms will make the skin there look a whole lot better. Give your skin a healthy, rosy glow by using an exfoliator at least twice a week when you're in the shower. Whether you choose one from the luxury body care ranges or a budget buy, you'll notice the difference immediately.**

## How does it work?

A therapist uses a hand-held machine that pumps out a stream of minute crystals on to the skin. These crystals, which act like super-exfoliators, are made of a hard material such as aluminium oxide or sodium bicarbonate, and gradually 'sandblast' away all the dead skin cells on the surface, smoothing out tiny lumps and bumps which together make the skin look uneven and patchy. The machine vacuums up the crystals and dead skin cells, leaving you with a pinky glow and smooth-as-satin thighs (or wherever).

Some of the newer machines operate with a diamond-tipped wand instead of shooting out a stream of particles, but they all have a similar effect. At the end of the treatment the therapist will often moisturise the targeted areas with a specialised lotion or cream to help protect the new skin. For best results a treatment about every eight weeks is recommended.

*Try another idea...*

**What you wear can make all the difference to whether anyone knows you've got cellulite or not. To avoid getting caught wearing the wrong trousers, turn to IDEA 17, *Be a mistress of disguise.***

The machines can operate at varying strengths and can remove just the surface layer of skin or go a bit deeper, depending on how comfortable it feels for the recipient.

## Is there pain with the gain?

Anyone who had microdermabrasion a few years ago might say a definite 'yes', but the technique has been refined since then and although it probably can't be called pleasant, it shouldn't be painful. It has been described by those who've had it as like fingernails lightly scratching the skin. Anyway, it's likely to be less uncomfortable on the bottom than it is on the face, where it's more commonly used, so you're getting off lightly, really.

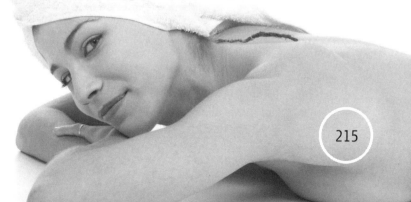

# Is it safe?

Therapists wielding these gadgets need to know what they are doing – they should move the machine evenly over the targeted areas to remove just the surface layer of skin (the stratum corneum) without damaging the deeper layers underneath.

Defining idea...

'*I want to have a good body, but not as much as I want dessert.*'
JASON LOVE

The skin may be red or pink afterwards, but this should only last a few hours. You do have to keep any 'new' skin that's exposed to the sun's rays (even if it's not particularly sunny) well protected with a high-factor sun cream. Apart from sensitivity to the sun, the skin will also be more sensitive to anything else you put on it, so follow the advice of the therapist about which products are safe to use.

# DIY microdermabrasion

If your budget doesn't run to a course of salon treatments, several mainstream cosmetics companies have come up with 'try this at home' versions. The kits usually contain a powerful exfoliant, some of which have aluminium oxide crystals similar to those used by the salon machines, and protective moisturisers to put on the skin afterwards. Some of the kits have a battery-powered gadget alternative to the salon machine for extra oomph, but the effects are still likely to be less noticeable than after a salon session.

**Tip** Whatever you do, make sure you follow the instructions carefully with any of these kits, so as not to overdo the treatment and end up looking like a boiled lobster (or worse).

# How did it go?

**Q: I really want to try microdermabrasion – I'd give anything for a baby-smooth bottom – but I'm not sure about these aluminium crystals. Isn't aluminium supposed to be bad for you?**

A: You've got a point. There has been some controversy about aluminium in various contexts and although it's used in certain body products, such as deodorants, some people are sensitive to it. The use of sodium bicarbonate (baking soda) crystals was developed as a safer alternative to aluminium oxide crystals – the salon therapist should be able to tell you what their machine uses before you book.

**Q: This sounds like a good treatment for just before you go on a beach holiday, doesn't it?**

A: No! The last thing you want to expose new skin to is the sun – UV rays cause enough damage to ordinary skin, let alone skin that's just had the top layer scraped off. If you want microdermabrasion in order to look better in a bikini (which is understandable, we know) you need to have the treatment at least a month before you go on holiday. And don't forget the high-factor sunscreen!

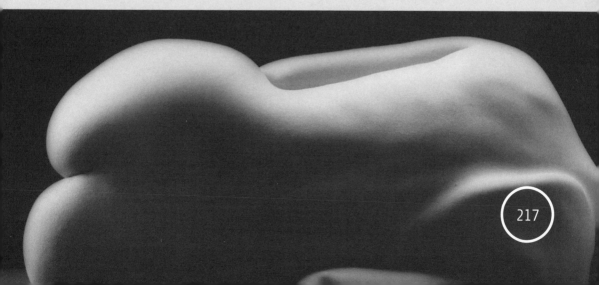

217

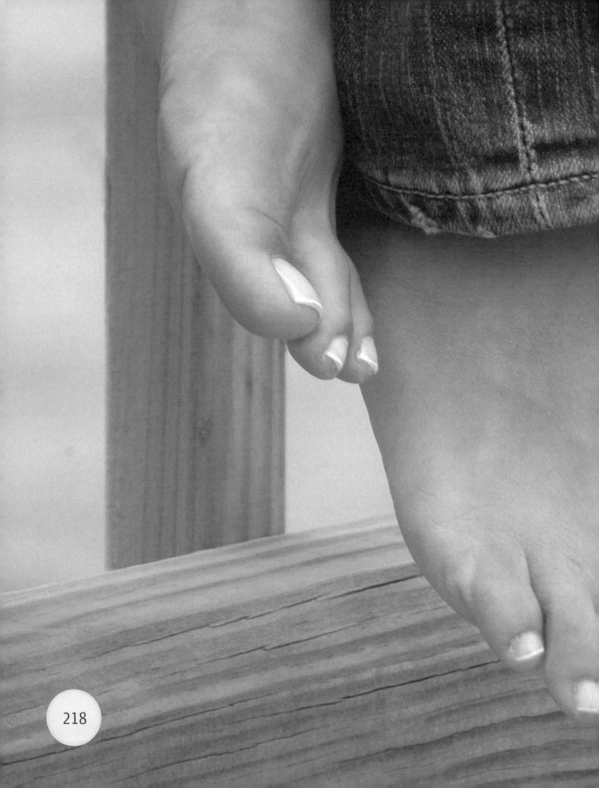

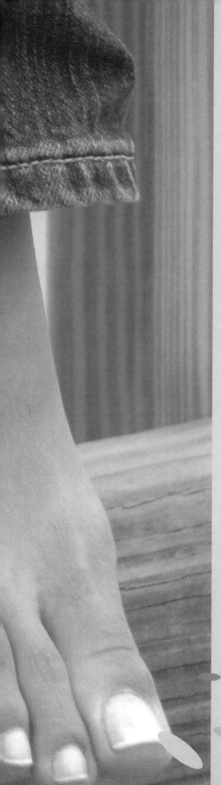

# 40

# Getting a leg up

**Walk your way to firmer, sexier legs – with a little help from MBTs, or Masai Barefoot Technology trainers.**

Can the type of shoes you wear really make a difference to the dimply stuff on your bottom? Here's the lowdown on the trainers nicknamed 'fatburners'.

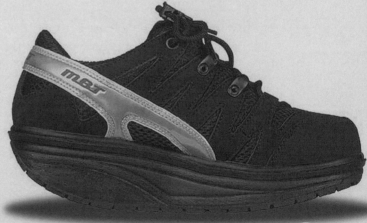

Sounds like a fairytale, doesn't it? You put on a pair of shoes and, as if by magic, your cellulite starts to disappear...Well, let's not get too carried away – you do have to actually walk in them. And first you have to learn how to walk in them. Their thick, curved soles give them a platform, and make you walk in a different way, so that your feet are 'rolling' rather than the heel absorbing most of the impact as it does with normal footwear.

Like many aids to reducing cellulite, these trainers were designed for their health benefits, with the inch loss to orange-peel thighs a welcome bonus. They were originally developed in the 1980s by a Swiss professor, Karl Muller, to help cure back and joint problems by correcting the posture and altering the load on the spine.

Now that their many benefits have been revealed, celebrities as well as sports professionals have had themselves fitted for a pair. Jemima Khan, Madonna, Gisele Bundchen, Sadie Frost and Zoe Ball have all been seen rolling along with a pair of MBTs on their feet, and glossy magazines such as *Vogue* have featured them.

> ### Here's an idea for you...
>
> **To get the maximum benefit from wearing MBTs you need to walk as much as you possibly can. So leave the car in the garage and walk to work/to the station/into town/to see friends. Carry your work shoes or evening Manolos with you and change when you get there – the longer you wear your MBTs the better the results. The extra exercise will help you lose inches and tone up your bottom even more.**

## How do they work?

The curved layers of the sole emulate walking on natural, uneven surfaces – which our bodies were designed to do – as opposed to the artificial hard and flat surfaces we mostly walk on today. This forces the body into a more upright posture and means you use muscle groups that are normally neglected. With better posture – think of a proud Masai warrior walking across an African plain – your back and joints are strengthened, circulation is improved and you even breathe more efficiently.

Because the body is working more efficiently and extra muscles are being used, more calories are being burned and weight loss is speeded up. MBTs improve muscle activation by 38%, so any workout is 38% more effective. Bottom and leg muscles are toned up more quickly – even while standing the muscles continue working to maintain a centre of balance.

*Try another idea...*

**It may be purely cosmetic, but keeping your skin well moisturised and nourished can make cellulite patches look a whole lot better. For tips on how to keep skin in tip top condition turn to IDEA 7, *Cream's crackers*.**

Losing excess fat on bottom and thighs means less cellulite. With improved muscle tone over the whole of the lower body, any remaining cellulite will be less visible, and more efficient circulation will boost blood supply to the skin tissues, further improving skin texture.

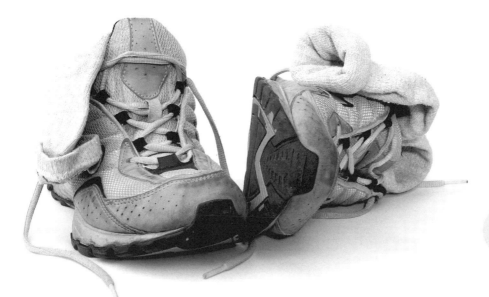

## What do they feel like?

MBTs take a bit of getting used to. The thick
layers of curved sole feel awkward at first because
they make you feel as if you're walking on an
uneven surface (that's the point). After wearing
them for the first time – usually for just half an
hour's walking – you'll feel as if your legs have
had a good workout (which they have) and may
ache a bit. But once you've got used to them it
feels like floating – some wearers can't bear to be parted from them.

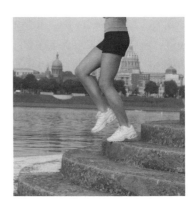

Other wearers have felt a burning sensation in their feet after walking in them. This
is due to the increased blood flow to the foot muscles and should disappear after a
few weeks. However, if it doesn't, the manufacturers advise a visit to your GP as it
could indicate some kind of vascular problem.

If you get backache after wearing them it's because the back muscles are getting used
to a different posture, and should settle down after a while. In fact, some MBT wearers
have reported a big improvement in their back problems, including lower back pain.

## The right fit to get fit

The big plus of MBTs is you don't have to change your daily routine at all to get any
of these benefits – you just put on a different pair of shoes. MBTs come in several
styles and colours and there's even an open-toed sandal for summer. They are not
much more expensive than high-quality 'normal' trainers, so whichever way you
look at it they are probably a worthwhile investment.

You can't buy MBTs mail order because they need to be properly fitted to make sure you are using them correctly. They come in slightly more varied sizing than standard footwear and need to fit snugly. The trained fitter will also give you a lesson in how to walk properly in them. There is now an international following and MBTs are becoming more easily available through sports shops and department stores. For prices and where to buy visit www.mbt-info.com. Roll on!

> Defining idea...
> **'A man's health can be judged by which he takes two at a time – pills or stairs.'**
> JOAN WELSH

## How did it go?

**Q: Can I use MBT trainers for all types of exercise?**

A: You can wear them every day for pretty much any exercise that you don't need specialised footwear for – jogging or running, the gym or exercise classes. You do need to get used to them first though, as the sensation is like walking on an uneven surface, so it's probably best not to put them on for the first time and go straight into a new step class.

**Q: I've just splashed out on a pair of MBTs. How long should I wear them for each day?**

A: You should only wear them for 30–45 minutes per day for the first week. Gradually add another 15–30 minutes per day every week, until you can wear them comfortably for more than two hours at a stretch. By this time your muscles will be attuned to them and you can start wearing them as much as you want – all day every day if you like.

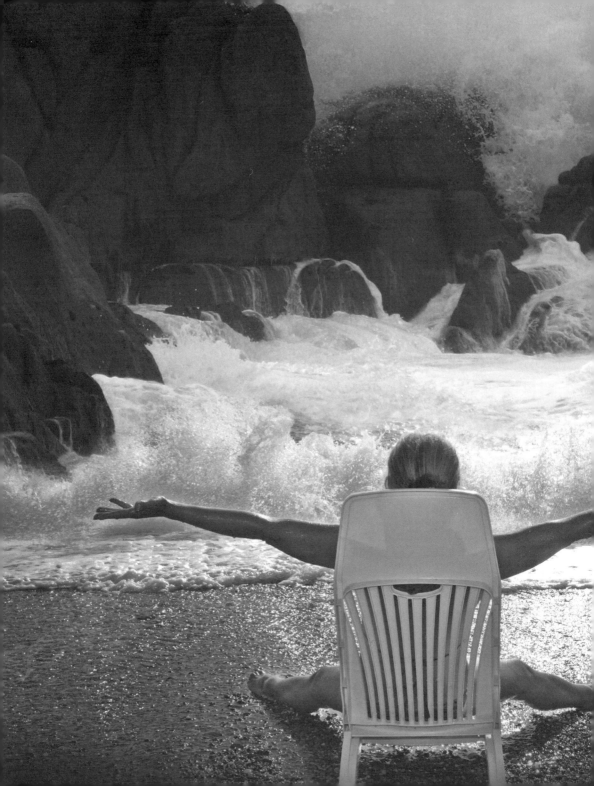

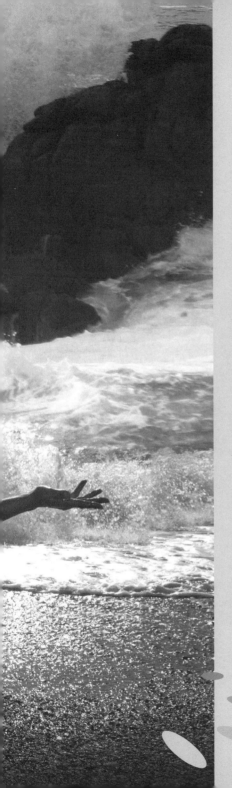

# 41

# Getting your sea legs

**Brace yourself for thalassotherapy – mineral-rich seawater feeds the skin and hot and cold water jets stimulate your circulation.**

If you're sick of cellulite, it's time you had more water. Don't worry,

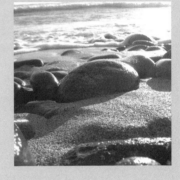

we're not going to suggest you start drinking ten glasses a day instead of six to eight (be honest, sometimes six is hard enough). This time it's water that goes straight to your thighs from the outside – seawater, to be precise.

'Thalasso' means 'sea' in Greek and thalassotherapy covers a whole range of different kinds of therapy involving seawater. You don't have to look far for evidence of the healing and curing powers of the sea – for a start, we know that salty seawater is loaded with minerals and can help heal skin wounds. And have you ever had a dip in the sea and not felt invigorated, refreshed and better all over?

The sea has therapeutic powers that are still not fully understood, but thalassotherapists are convinced it can help with a long list of problems, including cellulite. Why? Because the sea contains a virtual A–Z of minerals, from aluminium to zinc, which have a whole raft of beneficial effects on the skin and body. This potent mix includes minerals with antioxidant properties that have a detoxifying and anti-ageing effect, such as selenium (detoxifying), potassium (anti-ageing and helps regulate the body's fluid levels), magnesium and iodine (both good for metabolism), to mention just a handful.

The theory is that through regular soaks in seawater, or warm water with a concentrated mix of sea minerals added, some of these health-giving nutrients are absorbed into the body to help detoxify, diminish water retention, feed the skin and boost its production of new collagen. All of these are great in themselves, but they are all big pluses in the battle against cellulite too.

And that's before we get to the fun part – the water jets. Now, this is not a lying-down-being-pampered type of treatment, but invigorating? Say no more! Just strip

*Here's an idea for you...*
**Don't you think you deserve a treat? Book yourself a couple of days of anti-cellulite pampering at a spa that specialises in thalassotherapy treatments. The true definition of a thalassotherapy spa is that it is 300 m or less from the sea – so you get to spend some therapeutic time on the beach too.**

off (swimsuits are OK), brace yourself, and the therapist will train alternate hot and cold jets of water at your cellulite. The force of the jets is quite powerful (just think, the more powerful it is the more difference it could be making), but not painful – most people find it refreshing and say they feel fantastic afterwards.

The idea is that the force of the jets coupled with the extremes of temperature crank the circulation up a gear, and it is sluggish circulation that is linked to cellulite. To improve your cellulite you need your skin to be working at its optimum level. It needs to be fed nutrients and oxygen like any other organ in the body, and it's your blood circulation that brings all the goodies to the skin, whether that's the skin on your face or on your bottom. If the jets contain seawater so much the better, but if they contain plain water they should still have a circulation-boosting effect, though this would be called hydrotherapy rather than thalassotherapy.

*Try another idea...*
**Lying down and being massaged with fragrant oils sounds like pampering to us, but it's also a great ally in the war against crinkly thighs. Turn to IDEA 26, *Scents of a woman*.**

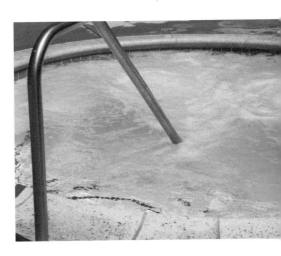

What the jets also do is stimulate the lymphatic system. The therapist trains the jets at the ankles first and moves up the body, in the correct sequence to encourage lymph drainage, which combats water retention and helps rid the body of waste products –two more ways to fight cellulite.

So where do you go for all this invigorating, cellulite-bashing water therapy? Long live the spa boom! Spas have really taken off all over the world in the past few years, which is good news for those of us with semolina bottoms. You'll find day spas in cities, spas at hotels and health farms, and for real bliss, luxury spas in exotic beachfront locations.

*Defining* idea...
**'The cure for anything is salt water: sweat, tears or the sea.'**
ISAK DINESEN

The French are mad keen on thalassotherapy and there are lots of spas along the coasts where you can have jets full of filtered seawater trained on you. Most other countries are not as far advanced with true thalassotherapy using real seawater. Spas in the UK, for instance, have not yet made the investment needed to get the seawater piped in, so they may use powdered sea minerals or add seaweed extracts to their baths and pools instead.

If you're heading to a spa, find out what other sea-based treatments they have and make the most of a combination of cellulite-reducing therapies. One to go for is a seaweed bodywrap, often suggested for immediately after water jet treatment. The more seawater treatments you can get, the more you'll feel like The Little Mermaid.

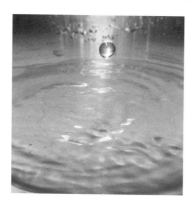
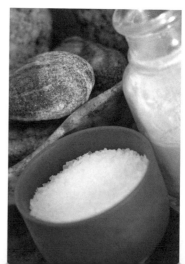

## How did it go?

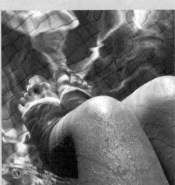

### Q: What about jet baths instead of showers? Do these work?

A: These have a similar effect. You sit in the hydro bath while strategically placed underwater jets are turned on in a specific sequence.

### Q: I've been having MLD (manual lymphatic drainage), which is a nice gentle massage, so how can this powerful water massage be doing the same job?

A: You're right, MLD is a gentle massage, but it is stimulating the lymph system in a different way. MLD concentrates on getting the lymph nodes (in the armpits, groin, neck, etc.) to open and close to get the system working more efficiently. Both treatments should have a similar effect though. So, gentle or rough? The choice is yours – it's a personal thing!

### Q: What else has the sea got to offer by way of cellulite treatment?

A: Some women battling dimpled thighs swear by anti-cellulite tea, a brew containing ingredients to boost circulation. It includes green tea, mint, lemon and fucus algae, the 'slimming seaweed', and is also said to be an appetite suppressant. What does it taste like? Well, if you're a fan of herbal teas, probably fine, if not then it may take a little getting used to. Find out more at www.thalgo.com.

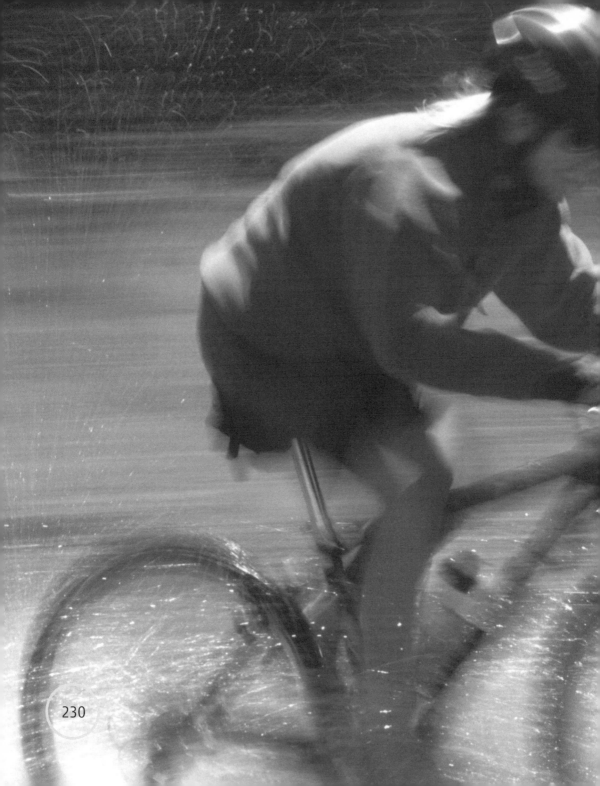

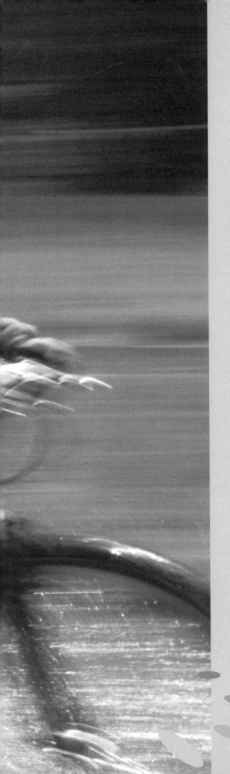

# 42

# Pedal power

**Cycling is great exercise for turning a spongy bottom into a pert rear of the year, and for toning and trimming both the back and front of the thighs, diminishing cellulite as you go. The only saddle bags will be the ones over your back wheel.**

Old-fashioned cycling exercises exactly the areas where cellulite accumulates — hips, bottom and thighs. But you can also try the space age cycle and vacuum treatment to target the dimples.

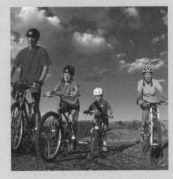

231

Have you got a bike in the back of the shed covered in cobwebs? Do you want to have less cellulite? Well, get your cycle shorts on and dust down your helmet – you have just discovered a new way to trim the dimply bits off your bottom that is easy, fun...and free!

As a powerful lower body workout, cycling is a great way to tone up your thigh muscles and gluteus maximus (those big muscles in your bottom). As an aerobic exercise it burns fat and calories (a substantial 400 calories an hour on the flat and more on hills), boosts circulation and is also a good cardiovascular workout for a healthy heart.

*Here's an idea for you...*

**Don't want to ride alone? Join a cycling club, discover different routes to ride and open up a whole new, fun side to your social life. And there will always be someone around to help you mend that puncture.**

You don't even have to allow any extra time in your week to fit in this particular cellulite-busting regime – just use it as your primary method of getting from A to B. Cycle to work if you possibly can, and jump on your bike to do errands or visit friends. And before you get in the car to go anywhere, get in the habit of asking yourself, 'Could I get there by bike?'

Like all exercise, cycling boosts circulation, which fights the build up of cellulite. The calorie burn gets rid of any excess fat on hips and bottoms, and the muscle sculpting leaves you with toned legs from your trim ankles to the tops of your thighs.

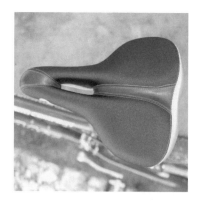

The trend for mountain biking has made cycling cool and in some areas opened up whole new networks of trails for riders. And there's mountains of stylish gear to choose from. Black Lycra padded cycling shorts can be surprisingly flattering, or you could disguise your cellulite in full-length, ankle-hugging stretch trousers with matching shirt – and don't forget the wraparound shades.

Get your friends out on some pub cycle rides or picnic rides at the weekends and turn improving your cellulite into a party. Just take it easy on the beer and cheese and onion crisps.

*Try another idea...*

**If the thought of taking to the road is a bit daunting (all that traffic!), then you might want to think of something you can do indoors. Time to cha-cha-cha. IDEA 46, *Dance with a stranger*, will show you how.**

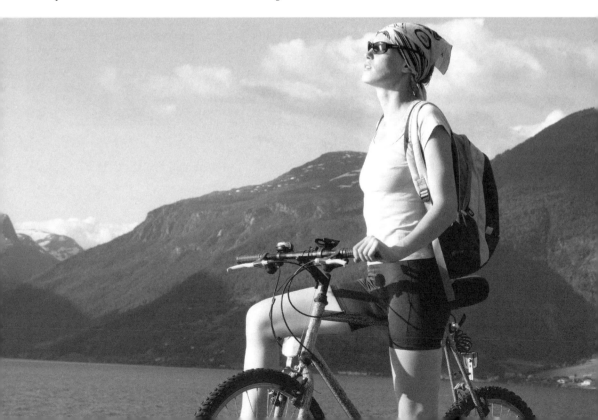

# Warm up before saddling up

Before and after you get on your bike, make sure you stretch your muscles, particularly those in the calf and thigh. Cycling can tend to shorten muscles – there's no built-in stretching as there would be in an exercise class – which can end up making you less flexible.

- Stretch the calf muscles by bending your left leg and placing both hands on your knee, at the same time placing your right heel on the floor with toes pointing upwards. Hold the stretch for 20–30 seconds and repeat with the other leg.

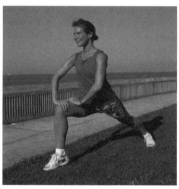

- Stretch the quad muscles at the front of your thigh by standing on one leg and bending the other one up behind you, holding on to your ankle – keep your knees together to maximise the stretch and count to 30. Repeat with the other leg.

- Stretch the backs of your legs by standing with your feet apart, keeping your legs straight and bending over to touch the ground – hold for 30 seconds.

**Now saddle up and head for the hills!**

# Try the cycle and suck method

There's a newish treatment for cellulite that looks like something out of a Woody Allen spoof sci-fi movie, but could get results. Called hypoxi-therapy, it combines cycling with vacuum suction (see what we mean?) You sit on an exercise bike and pedal away, but from the waist down you are enclosed in a futuristic 'slimming pod' vacuum chamber. While your pedal power burns the calories, the vacuum's sucking action increases the blood supply to your below-the-belt cellulitey areas, accelerating fat and cellulite breakdown.

This does take a bit of effort – one tester described it as similar to cycling through sand – and money (as much as a decent new bike!), but there have been some satisfied customers. One woman lost half a stone and about 45% of her cellulite. Find out more at www.hypoxitraining.com.

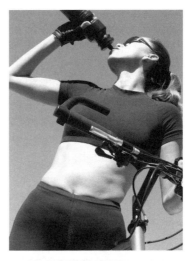

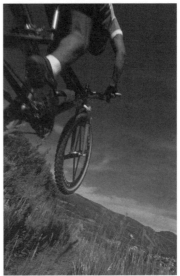

## Spin those wheels

Check out 'spinning' classes at your local gym or health club. These are the classes where everyone sits on fixed exercise bikes with the resistance at quite a high setting, pedalling like crazy to loud music, changing positions and speeds according to the class leader. Hard work but fun, spinning can burn as much as 500 calories in 40 minutes, and if you join in regularly, your legs cannot fail to get more toned, sculpted and slimmer.

## How did it go?

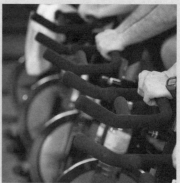

**Q: I haven't got a bike. Will doing bicycling exercises lying on the floor in my sitting room work just the same?**

A: Not quite. Cycling is weight-bearing exercise – you are pressing down on the pedals and using muscles in the legs in a different way to lying on the floor and cycling in the air. Bicycling exercises on the floor are usually designed to strengthen the stomach muscles rather than the thighs and bottom.

**Q: Are static exercise bikes as good as the real thing?**

A: They're pretty close, but you won't get as varied a workout for your leg and buttock muscles because you won't encounter different terrain – hills, slopes and so on. You'll also lose out on the health and feel-good benefits of spending time in the great outdoors.

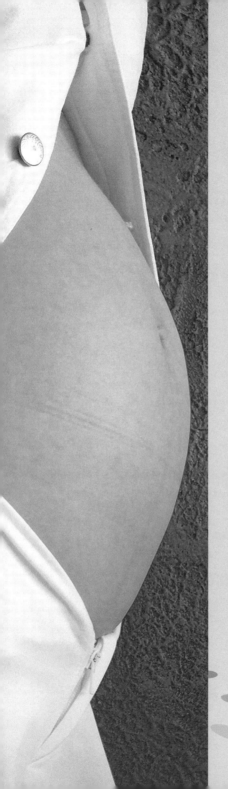

# 43

# Ladykillers

**The higher your levels of oestrogen, the more likely you are to have cellulite. (Who said life was fair?) We have strategies to help.**

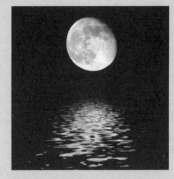

Fact 1: Women get cellulite, men don't. Fact 2: Women have different hormones to men — we have lots of oestrogen in our bodies, men don't. Fact 3: Many women complain that cellulite gets worse when they are pregnant or soon afterwards — a time when oestrogen increases.

237

It's no surprise, then, that many of the boffins who have been trying to work out what causes crinkly bottoms favour the theory that it has a lot to do with female hormones.

Oestrogen is also linked to fat and the way it is stored in the body. If women put on weight their bodies produce more oestrogen, and those with high levels of oestrogen tend to have extra fat around their bottom, hips and thighs – i.e. they're pear shaped.

If this sounds like you, look on the bright side. You are a fertility goddess. Research has revealed that pear-shaped women are more fertile than their snake-hipped sisters. You can probably blame it all on the cavewomen. Mrs Flintstone needed to store enough fat on her body not only to survive lean times herself, but support a pregnancy and create the next generation.

*Here's an idea for you...*
**Try sprinkling linseed over your muesli, drinking soya milk and eating soya desserts, and buying Burgen soya and linseed bread. These foods all contain phytoestrogens. If you're genuinely pear-shaped you should include lots of these plant hormones in your diet, as they have a balancing effect on your oestrogen-dependent fatty deposits.**

Who knows – maybe cellulite saved the human race!

Oestrogen also encourages fluid retention, which some experts believe is key to causing cellulite, with water trapped between fat cells.

## Low-fat, low-fad diet

You can't really control how much oestrogen you've got or where your body stores fat, but you can give it less fat to store. If you have the sort of body that seems to hang on to every molecule of fat as if it was expecting a famine at any moment, following a diet that's healthy but low fat makes sense.

When it comes to food choices, knowledge is power. You may already have a good grasp of which foods are naturally high, medium or low in fat, but if you don't, it's worth absorbing as much information as you can – it'll make shopping, cooking and choosing from menus so much quicker and easier!

> ### Try another idea...
> **Massage is a great way to boost your circulation, encourage lymphatic drainage and de-stress – all of which should have a positive effect on your cellulite. But you don't have to book a session at a salon. For how to self-massage at home turn to IDEA 20, *Gold fingers*.**

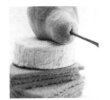 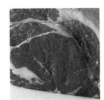 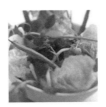 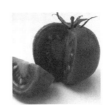

There is no need to buy any special 'diet' foods, or follow specific diet regimes unless you want to. Simple strategies such as cutting down on the obvious high-fat foods such as cheese, butter, full-fat milk, bacon and burgers (make sure you're getting your protein and calcium elsewhere) and piling on the fruit and vegetables, which have massive health benefits anyway, can make a big difference.

We all need some fat in our diets, but most of us are getting much more than we need. Part of the problem is our reliance on ready meals, and stuff in packets, cans and boxes – processed foods are often higher in fats than we realise. The ideal solution, and the one that's the healthiest for all of us, is to eat more fresh food and cook more, rather than opening packets and shoving the contents in the microwave. That way, at least we know what we're eating.

Before you yell 'I don't have time to cook!', remember that we've been fooled into thinking we don't have time by a rapacious convenience food industry. How much time does it really take to throw together a salad or rustle up a stir fry? (Despite it's name, stir fry uses hardly any fat – so invest in a wok!)

Finally, beware of buying low-fat versions of foods such as yoghurts – these often have lower fat but more sugar, which won't do your cellulite any good either.

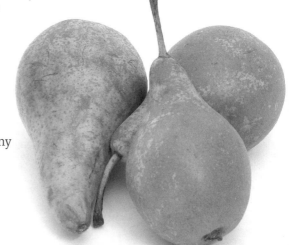

# Burn off the fat

If you're a high-oestrogen, pear-shaped kind of girl, get those legs moving with speed-walking, cycling or running to both burn off fat quickly and tone the whole of your lower body. If you've got a big bottom, this will help turn it from a wobbly blancmange into a high, sexy firm globe that will make men's eyes swivel – think J-Lo!

If you've got a bottom-heavy figure, you can help balance this out by doing some upper-body exercise as well to tone and develop the muscles in your arms, back and chest. This could be the moment to dust down that gym membership card and get some advice on the best upper-body exercise machines for you. If you're happier outdoors, Nordic walking will give you the double whammy of exercising both upper and lower body at the same time (www.nordicwalking.com).

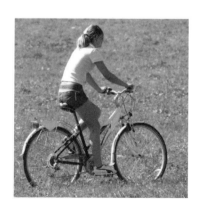

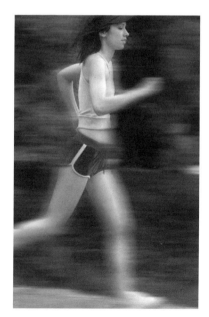

## How did it go?

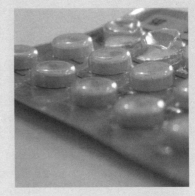

**Q: It could be a coincidence, but I first noticed I had cellulite after I started taking the Pill. Can this have made a difference?**

A: Since the Pill contains a synthetic form of oestrogen, yes it could. It may not make a difference to everyone though, and no one knows how much of a difference. You could try coming off it and see for yourself, but remember that the Pill is one of the most reliable forms of contraception!

**Q: I am in my late forties and have hit the menopause, so my oestrogen levels must be dropping. Does that mean my cellulite will automatically improve?**

A: Oops, sorry, not necessarily. Life is cruel sometimes, and unfortunately one of the effects of ageing is that it's not very helpful to cellulite. The skin loses collagen as we get older, and the connective tissues around the fat underneath the skin become less flexible, pulling against it and resulting in more bulges and dimples. Ageing skin can start to look like crepe paper too, particularly if it's dehydrated, making cellulite look worse. So any gains there might have been from less oestrogen are likely to be cancelled out. But all is not lost! Keeping slim, fit and healthy and drinking plenty of water will go a long way to improving your cellulite, whatever your age.

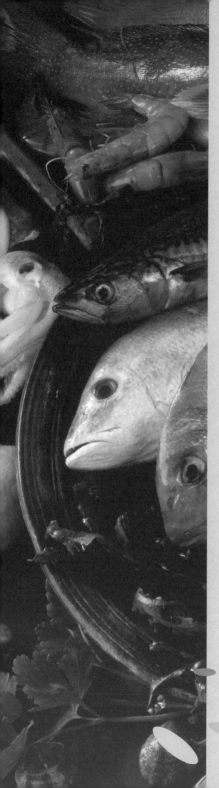

# 44

# A la carte cellulite-busting

**Revamp your eating habits to smooth out those dimples. Here are some quick, easy recipes for low-fat meals that anyone can try, containing foods that will help improve your cellulite.**

Can't cook, won't cook? Of course you can. It's easy and quick, and cooking with fresh ingredients means you get more of the vitamins and nutrients that help keep dimply flesh at bay.

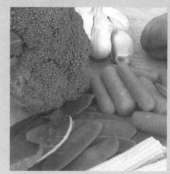

The big principles of eating to beat cellulite are having more fresh and fewer processed foods and ready-made meals, loading up with fruit and veg, cutting down on fat and avoiding too much salt. Oh, and try not to over-eat. Cellulite is fat and fat is what you get when you eat more calories than you can use up in energy. Not rocket science, but some foods do more than others to help you diminish your cellulite. These are the foods that help boost circulation, sending nutrients to improve skin condition; help strengthen tissues around fat cells to stop them bulging out; diminish water retention; and assist the body's natural waste-disposal systems.

Here's an idea
for you...
**Have one or two days a week when you eat only raw foods to spring-clean your system and help the detoxification process. Think enormous platefuls of all your favourite salad ingredients, loads of fruit, snacks of nuts and freshly squeezed juices. You'll fill up with first-class nutrients – raw fruit and vegetables retain more vitamins than those that have been cooked – and lose weight too.**

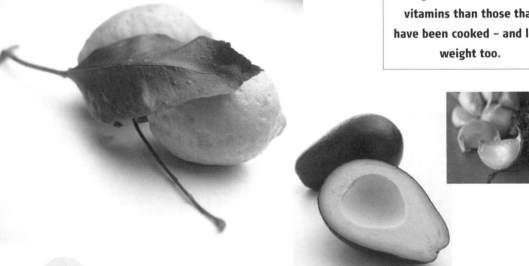

To give you a helping hand here are some anti-cellulite foods, followed by easy-peasy recipes with an emphasis on fresh veg to get you started. All recipes should serve two; adjust the quantities for fewer or more people.

**Onions** – good for circulation and detoxing, high in antioxidants that help improve the skin.

**Garlic** – ditto, plus helpful for metabolism.

**Oranges** – top for vitamin C, which keeps connective tissue between fat cells under the skin strong and supple.

**Blueberries**, **raspberries**, **strawberries** and other blue or red berries are high in antioxidants, which are good for your skin and lymph system, and vitamin C.

**Apples** – good source of pectin fibre for detoxing, potassium for fluid-flushing, vitamin C for skin.

**Bananas** – potassium for anti-ageing and fluid retention, fibre for waste disposal.

**Grapefruit** – vitamin C, fibre, detoxifying.

**Tomatoes** – vitamin C, antioxidants, good for skin.

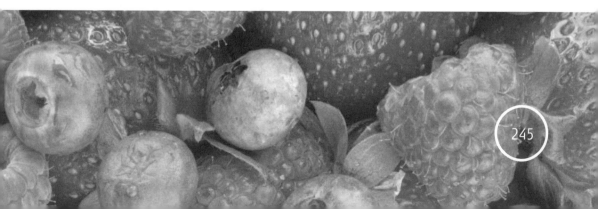

**Broccoli** – helps avoid water retention, good for detox, antioxidants for skin.

**Spinach** – good for circulation (vitamin K) and skin, anti-ageing.

**Celery** – helps avoid water retention.

**Red peppers** – high in vitamin C and antioxidants.

**Carrots** – detoxifying, antioxidants for skin.

**Chicken and turkey** – lean protein for collagen production, helping strengthen connective tissue around fat cells.

**White fish** – high protein, low fat.

**Salmon**, **tuna** and other oily fish, for omega-3 fatty acids that improve skin.

**Eggs** – low-fat protein, good for skin.

**Tofu** – low-fat protein.

**Spices** – circulation boosters include cayenne pepper and chillies.

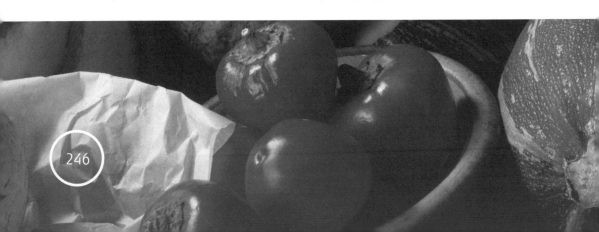

# Root veg in tomato and herb sauce

You can throw in whatever root vegetables you have for this; the potato and sweet potato make it filling.

## What you need

Two carrots
3–4 potatoes
1 medium sweet potato
1 large courgette, sliced
1 onion, finely chopped
1 clove garlic, crushed
1 400 g can chopped tomatoes
1 dessert spoon tomato puree
1 teaspoon fresh torn mixed herbs (e.g. thyme, oregano, basil)
2 tbsp extra virgin olive oil
Black pepper

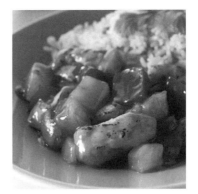

*Try another idea...*

**It's not just the fat in your diet that you need to watch. IDEA 16, *There's a rat in the kitchen*, has more useful food advice.**

Peel and chop up carrot, potato and sweet potato into bite-size chunks, put in boiling water for 10 minutes. While veg are cooking, heat oil in large heavy-bottomed pan with lid and cook onion and garlic for few minutes to soften and brown, then add courgette and cook for 5 minutes. Add tomatoes, tomato puree, herbs and black pepper, simmer for 2 minutes. Drain veg and add to other ingredients in pan, stir and simmer for 5 minutes and serve.

*The recipes in this idea are for two.*

# Chicken or tofu stir-fry with noodles

You'll need a wok (a good investment), and you can adjust quantities of veg to suit.

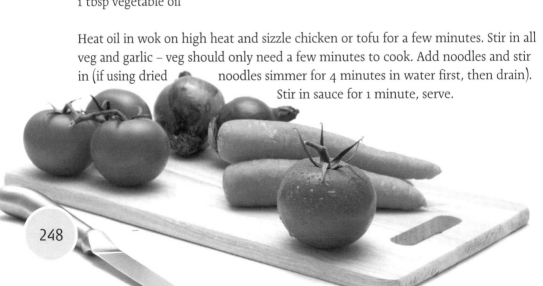

**What you need**
1 red and green pepper, cut into strips
1 clove garlic, crushed
1 carrot, cut into strips
Handful shredded spinach or cabbage
Handful broccoli florets
Handful beanshoots
(or if pushed for time buy a bag of pre-prepared stir-fry veg)
Noodles for two (fresh or dried)
1 chicken fillet, diced small, or equivalent amount of tofu, diced
1 packet chow mein stir-fry sauce (you're allowed the occasional packet!)
1 tbsp vegetable oil

Heat oil in wok on high heat and sizzle chicken or tofu for a few minutes. Stir in all veg and garlic – veg should only need a few minutes to cook. Add noodles and stir in (if using dried noodles simmer for 4 minutes in water first, then drain). Stir in sauce for 1 minute, serve.

# Onion and pepper omelette

Serve with lightly cooked broccoli and carrots.

**What you need**

2 left-over boiled potatoes, chopped
1 red pepper, diced
1 onion, finely chopped
3 eggs
Dash of milk or soya milk
Black pepper
2 tbsp vegetable oil

Heat oil in frying pan or omelette pan and cook
onion and pepper until soft; meanwhile beat eggs
in a bowl and add dash of milk and black pepper.
Add chopped potato to pan, cook for a few
minutes then pour egg mixture into pan. Shake
pan while cooking to avoid sticking, and turn
omelette when one side cooked. Serve when
underneath side cooked.

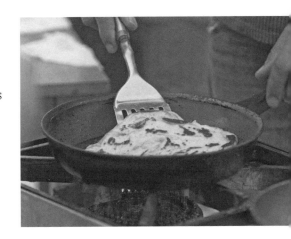

Defining idea...

'*Some things you have to do
every day. Eating seven
apples on Saturday night
instead of one a day just
isn't going to get the job
done.*'

JIM ROHN, entrepreneur and
motivational speaker

# And don't stop there!

Have fun experimenting with other easy veg-based dishes such as oven-roasted veg,
or vegetable chilli (chilli con carne without the carne), or make your own simple,
fast pasta sauce by gently frying onions, red pepper and garlic, then adding chopped
tomatoes and herbs. Cooking from scratch may be messy in the kitchen, but it's
fun, sociable and can be faster than sticking a ready meal in the oven.

249

## How did it go?

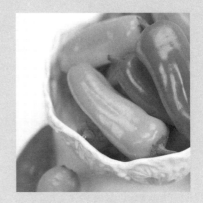

**Q: Sounds like I'd be better off being a vegetarian as far as shifting cellulite goes. Should I give this a try?**

A: Only if it means you're going to eat a lot more fresh fruit and veg – despite massive health campaigns most of us still don't get enough, especially vegetables. But you also need plenty of protein to produce new collagen to help skin keep cellulite under control, and most people find it easier to get protein from meats and fish.

**Q: What can I eat when I just don't have time to cook anything at all?**

A: Grab a carton of chunky vegetable or other veg-based fresh soup and stick it in the microwave. Not as good as fresh veg, but soup with lots of different ingredients is a good way of getting a high number of nutrients fast.

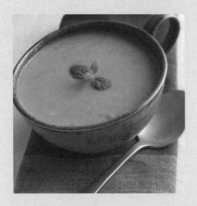

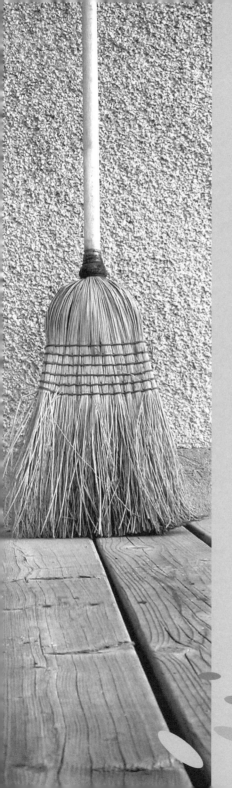

# 45

# Waste disposal

**Follow short-term detox cleansing regimes to help the liver get rid of waste products – including those that could increase your cellulite.**

*Glowing skin, weight loss, flat stomach and less obvious cellulite could all be possible if you regularly give your body a good old spring clean.*

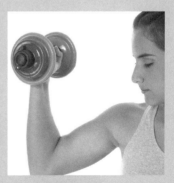

Had a run of parties and been forced to eat salty snacks? Had a bit of a thing about cake lately? Or just fallen off your healthy-eating wagon? Whatever, a short period of treating your body like a temple will help get you back on track. We're not talking about fasting or any other extreme detox measure, more a 'back to basics' approach and simple ideas to encourage your body to cleanse itself.

Let's get one thing straight, though. Detoxing won't magically melt away cellulite. Although a lot has been written about toxic build up as a cause of cellulite, the jury is still out, with opinion among those involved in studying and treating cellulite varying widely on this one.

Here's an idea
for you...

Freshly liquidised fruit and vegetable juices and smoothies are especially good for detoxing because the less energy your body needs to digest food, the more it will have to cleanse your system of toxins. Try to have as many liquid lunches (no, not that type) and breakfasts as you can, and if you haven't got a juicer, invest in one. Fresh juices are also an easy way of making sure you get your five portions of fruit and veg a day.

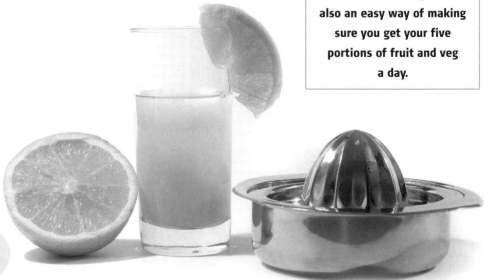

It's certainly true that the body has its own natural detoxifier – the liver – which will break down harmful substances from food, drink or other sources. But why not give it a helping hand? Regular stints of cutting out excess sugar, fats and processed foods, replacing alcohol and caffeine with water, and giving your poor old bod a well-earned rest from the daily onslaught of chemicals can only be a good thing.

Try another idea...

It's not always easy to eat the right things, but a better diet will show in your skin. IDEA 44, *A la carte cellulite-busting*, will give you some pointers to better eating.

After all, it's often the combination of low-nutrition, additive-laden foods, too much salt resulting in fluid retention, excess sugar leading to insulin release which in turn encourages fat storage, dehydration, and the dreaded smoking (you're not still doing that, are you?) that conspires to keep us cellulite-ridden. While genetics often plays a part, all of these are enemies to smooth, slender thighs.

So try a simple, calming and restorative detox strategy of between two and five days. It doesn't have to involve complex recipes, total deprivation or wallet-slimming stays at health farms. Just be kind to your body and simplify, simplify, simplify. Back this up with body care and anti-cellulite strategies such as dry skin brushing, massage, exfoliation and moisturising to give your skin a healthy glow.

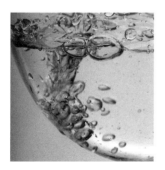
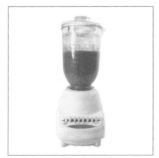
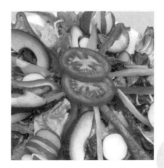

## Two to five day detox regime

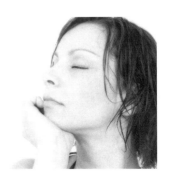

- Ditch the alcohol and caffeine and drink only water, herbal teas or fresh fruit and vegetable juices.

- Make sure you drink six glasses of water a day, to help your kidneys dilute and eliminate waste products.

- Ban sugar, including chocolate (a few days won't kill you).

- Ban processed ready-made foods.

- Cut down salt – no more than 6 g per day.

- Avoid saturated animal fats.

- Eat plenty of fruit and vegetables, as fresh as you can find. Apart from all the nutritional and antioxidant benefits, the fibre keeps your waste disposal system moving.

- Eat fruit and veg raw if possible, as salads, crudités or plates of cut fruit.

- Try to eat only organic produce, so you get the nutritional benefit as well as avoiding toxic pesticides.

- Include bananas because they are filling, potassium-rich (good for balancing your body's fluid levels), great energy boosters and full of fibre.

- Go veggie, and eat plenty of nuts, pulses and wholegrains or get high-quality protein from fresh fish, or organic chicken or eggs.

■ Try to avoid stress, especially if you're the sort of girl who wants to comfort eat when you're under pressure.

■ Walk, run or cycle in fresh air – get as far away from pollution as you can.

■ Create a calming, feel-good atmosphere at home with scented candles and low light.

■ Go to bed early and get lots of restorative sleep. If you need to, use relaxation tapes or a warm bath to get you off to dreamland.

Detoxing your body is good for your soul, too. Higher energy levels will make you feel more positive and motivated to get out there and do whatever it takes to zap your cellulite for good.

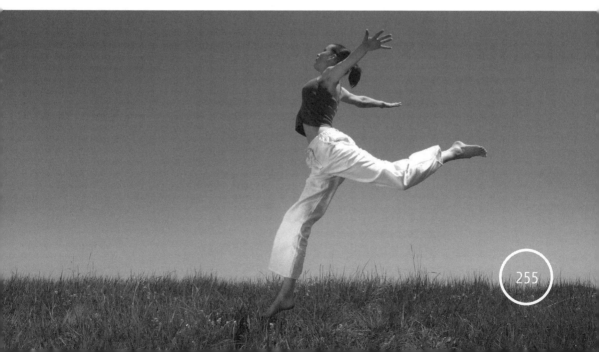

255

# How did it go?

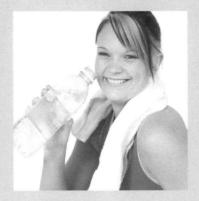

### Q: I'm pregnant. Can I still detox?

A: No. The baby needs a steady supply of nutrients from all the food groups, including protein, fats and carbohydrate. Just concentrate on eating healthily, including lots of fruit and veg.

### Q: I've tried eating loads of raw fruit and vegetables but it plays havoc with my digestion. Any ideas?

A: Some people do have a problem digesting raw fruit and vegetables. Try gently steaming your vegetables rather than boiling them – the lighter the cooking method, the better your chance of hanging on to those vital nutrients and antioxidants. And how about trying stewed fruit, such as plums or rhubarb. It's quick and easy: just add a small amount of water in a saucepan and simmer for a few minutes – experiment to get the consistency you like. (No, you *don't* need to add sugar.) Mix the stewed fruit with plain yoghurt for a delicious, healthy breakfast.

### Q: Isn't grapefruit meant to be good for detoxifying?

A: Yes, some people swear by it. Grapefruit is one of those 'superfoods' that can do everything. It contains pectin (which helps eliminate toxins), it helps boost your immunity and it has loads of vitamin C. Eating grapefruit before meals is also believed to take the edge off your appetite. The pink varieties are sweeter if you don't like too much tang first thing in the morning.

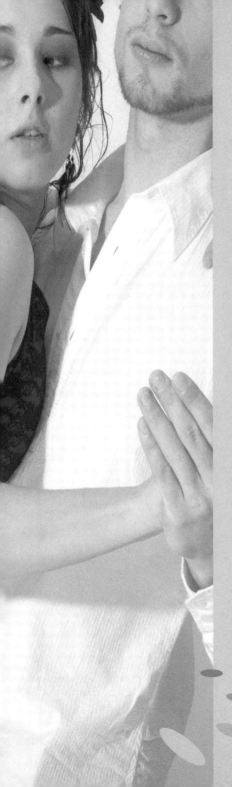

# 46

# Dance with a stranger

**Or by yourself. Well, have you ever seen a dancer with cellulite? From ballet to salsa, there'll be a dance exercise class that's right for you.**

Why shouldn't exercise be fun? As well as lifting your bottom, dance

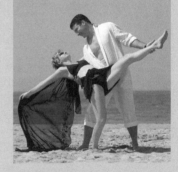

lifts your spirits too.

If someone told you you could reduce your cellulite by doing something that's fun, sociable, makes you feel good and can only be done while listening to great music, you'd jump at it, wouldn't you? Dancing is all of that and more. It's fantastic exercise for the whole body, but especially for the lower body – calves, thighs, bottom and stomach all get a really good workout.

In fact, dancing is probably one of the most undervalued forms of exercise there is. When we decide we want to get fit, lose weight or tone up we tend to head for the gym or start jogging. But joining a dance class could give us the same fitness level and help us drop a dress size, while having much more fun and learning something new.

And, if you can find the dance and music that does it for you, because it's exciting and fun instead of a chore, you'll never miss a session.

**Tip** As dancing is a form of exercise, always warm up before a class to avoid injuries.

## Ballet for grown-ups

You can always tell when you meet someone who has been a ballet dancer. They hold themselves upright, they are slim and graceful – even if they are eighty years old. You may not have much chance of becoming the next Darcey Bussell or Sylvie Guillem, but if you start ballet classes now you'll get all the benefits of better posture, flexibility, strength, stamina and better muscle tone.

### Here's an idea for you...

If you're single, make sure you choose a class where you have to dance with a partner. It takes two to tango, waltz or ballroom, and meeting someone new will give you an added incentive to dance your cellulite away – before he gets a chance to see it.

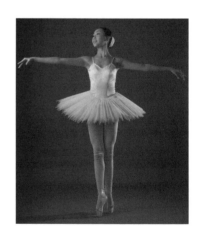

Ballet classes for adults have nothing to do with pink tutus and everything to do with developing a strong, lithe body. (Well, who wouldn't want the body of a ballerina?) The moves stretch and lengthen the muscles rather than add muscle bulk, to help create a lean, streamlined shape. Just about every ballet position tones and shapes your legs and bottom, from *pliés* (bending at the knees while keeping your back straight) to pirouettes.

*Try another idea...*

**If you take up dancing, you'll need all the oxygen you can get. And if you need another reason to give up smoking, IDEA 37, *Smoke gets in your eyes*, gives the lowdown on cigarettes and cellulite.**

If you have cellulite or wobbly bits on your inner thighs, ballet is the dance for you. Because the legs are so often in a 'turned out' position (toes pointing left and right instead of forwards), it's fantastic for the inner thighs. Just standing in a basic ballet position with your heels together and toes apart starts to work the backs of the legs and thighs. And moves such as the arabesque, when you lift a leg up at an angle that really squeezes the gluteus maximus, are just what a wobbly bottom needs.

If you're a total beginner you're unlikely to be doing *grands jetés* (big leaps) across the studio floor; you're more likely to be doing exercises at the barre. The emphasis is on sculpting the body rather than aerobics, although it will still help you lose any excess flab.

The other big plus with ballet is the arm movements that go with every new step you learn – great for flabby upper arms.

Once you know the moves you can practice at home in between classes: if done regularly enough you should start to notice a subtle change in your body shape within just a few weeks. And seeing your reflection in those floor-length studio mirrors is an added incentive not to head for the biscuit barrel when you get home.

# Assume the plié position

Try this basic version of the classic ballet exercise at home for the inner thighs (and bottom, quads and calves):

- Place your feet about shoulder width apart and turn your toes outwards to the sides.

- Hold your arms slightly rounded with hands curved towards each other below your waist.

- Breathe in and, as you breathe out, bend your knees as much as is comfortable, and lift your arms out to the sides to shoulder height, elbows slightly bent.

- Return to the starting position and repeat.

Do just a few *pliés* at first and gradually build up as your muscles become stronger.

# Sexy salsa

Latin American salsa is fast, fun and sexy and it can give you a real high. It's a close dance with a partner and the fact that 'salsa' means 'sauce' in Spanish says it all. With all that twisting and turning, stomping and leg kicking, it really works the bottom, legs, waist and hips.

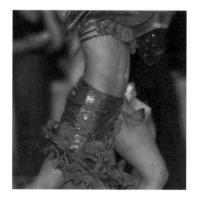

There's now such a huge enthusiasm for salsa that you shouldn't have too much trouble finding a class, and no, you don't have to bring a dance partner. Swapping partners and dancing with different people is part of the fun. But if you're worried about having two left feet, check out one of the 'how to salsa' DVDs that show you easy steps for beginners to give you a head start.

To get real benefits from any exercise you've got to do it regularly, which is where salsa fans win: it's so addictive there's even a group called 'salsaholics'...

## Street dance

If you really want to burn fat to reduce your cellulite zones, sign up for some of the more hot and happening dance classes known as 'street' dance. This is the kind of dance you see in pop videos and commercials, so if you've ever fancied yourself as a pop princess, here's your chance.

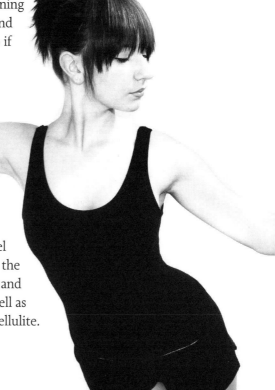

Classes can be a mix of different styles such as hip-hop or jazz – anything goes as long as it's funky, lively and fun.

These are some of the most aerobic dance classes there are (talk to the teacher about your fitness level first before signing up), and aerobic dance is one of the fastest ways to lose excess baggage around the hips and thighs. It gives the circulation a sure-fire boost as well as the metabolism, which helps in the battle against cellulite.

## How did it go?

**Q: Salsa sounds great but I'm only moderately fit and I don't want to look an idiot. Aren't the moves a bit complicated too?**

A: The steps are not particularly difficult; there are some complicated flourishes if you want to learn them but you'll always start off with simpler movements when you're a beginner. You don't need to be fantastically fit to salsa dance either – although it's high tempo you remain relatively stationary, with a lot of the movements almost 'on the spot'.

**Q: I'd love to join a dance class but I can't commit to making it to the sessions every week. What about videos and DVDs?**

A: There are lots of DVDs and videos that can teach you dance steps, but the best to use at home for tightening up wobbly thighs and reducing cellulite are those that are a combination of dance and fitness video/DVD. New York City Ballet, for instance, have produced DVDs based on ballet moves but with more aerobic exercises included. Sarah Jessica Parker of *Sex and the City* fame is a fan.

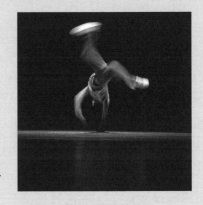

Defining idea...

'**Work like you don't need the money. Love like you've never been hurt. Dance like nobody's watching.**'
MARK TWAIN

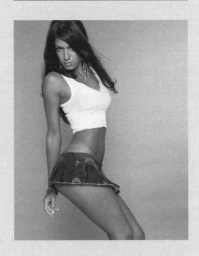

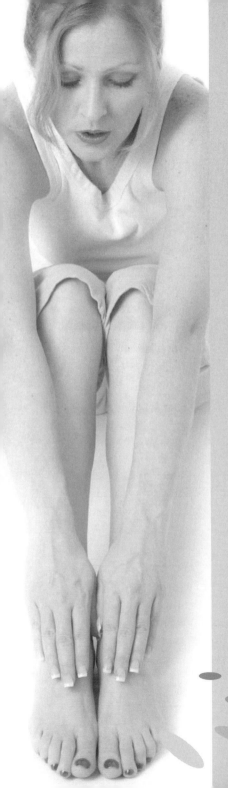

## 47

# Bend it, stretch it

**Follow the deep-stretching technique pioneered by movement and dance expert Marja Putkisto, to boost circulation and lymph drainage in the legs and smooth out cellulite.**

Deep breathing and deep stretching are the keys to the Putkisto method, originally created to improve flexibility, posture and energy. But its devotees — including people from the world of dance and sport — have noticed a reduction in cellulite, which could be due to better circulation and increased lymph flow.

Pilates teacher Marja Putkisto started to develop the Putkisto method twenty years ago, when she realised that many of us – herself included – are unable to stretch our muscles enough to allow our bodies to work properly.

She realised that our muscles get tight and are shortened from spending too much time sitting on our bottoms (sound familiar?). Our ribcages sink, the diaphragm pump can't work properly and circulation is permanently decreased and lymph flow restricted. Both circulation and lymph drainage have often been cited as keys to the cellulite mystery.

Here's an idea for you...
**Breathing deeply, so the air reaches the bottom of your lungs and not just the top, and slow, deep stretches that you hold for a couple of minutes have a brilliant de-stressing effect when you do them together. You may even become so laid back that you'll stop worrying about your cellulite altogether...**

Done regularly, the deep stretching helps lengthen the muscles and sort out body alignment and posture. You can't do the deep stretching properly without the deep breathing, which creates a natural rhythm, helping you time the stretches. Deep breathing gets more oxygen into the system, improving circulation and helping eliminate the toxins which could also contribute to cellulite.

One big advantage of this technique is that you don't have to spend any money. You can learn the method and do it any time you like in the comfort of your own sitting-room. But if you want to know more, Marja's method is fully explained, with lots more exercises for different parts of the body and a four-week programme, in her book *The Body Lean and Lifted: Stretch Yourself Slim in 30 Days.*

So, want to give it a go? When you're doing these exercises you need to use your mind as well and concentrate on feeling the different muscle groups in the body, so take your time. Once you've practised a few times it'll get easier.

Do this sequence of stretches to improve cellulite four or five times a week. To get maximum benefits, make sure you eat healthily (no junk food of course), drink plenty of water and walk 20 minutes a day.

*Try another idea...*

**After all this stretching and bending, fancy a pleasantly pulsing, electrical massage where you lie down and don't do a thing? Ionithermie exercises the muscles around your bottom and thighs for you. Find out more by turning to IDEA 3, *Shock treatment*.**

## Step 1: Lizard stretch to lengthen muscles around hips and pelvis

- Kneel on the floor, bend the right leg to create a 90-degree angle in front of your body with the foot flat on the floor.

- Extend your back leg behind you, staying upright with your chest lifted, and tilt your tailbone towards your navel.

- Rotate your back leg from your hip joint slightly inwards.

- Breathe in through the nose, focusing on the air reaching the lowest part of your lungs, then exhale slowly through your mouth, creating the stretch at the end of the outbreath.

- Continue the stretch with the flow of your breathing, applying more body weight through your pelvis to increase the stretch, for 2–5 minutes.

- Repeat on the other side.

265

## Step 2: Bow stretch to increase lymph flow

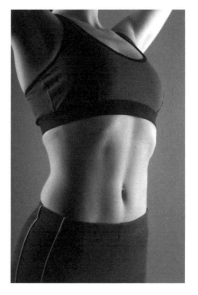

- Stand with your right side near a wall. Place the heel of your right foot on top of your left foot.

- Lift right elbow upwards, rotating it from the shoulder, and place the palm of that hand against the wall.

- Drop your head towards your left shoulder.

- Place your left hand on the right side of your lower ribcage.

- Focus on increasing the space between your pelvis and ribcage, creating a 'bow' stretch by bending your supporting leg and arm.

- Breathe in deeply through your nose to expand the side you are stretching.

- As you breathe out through your mouth, the rise of the diaphragm lifts your ribs away from your pelvis.

- Pause, and then further separate your ribs from your pelvis by dropping your weight towards your waistline (be careful not to lean on your hand).

- Continue the stretch with the flow of your breathing for 2–5 minutes.

  - Repeat on the other side.

# Step 3: Fishtail stretch for pelvis and thighs

- Lie on the floor on your right side and support your head with your right arm.

- Turn your tailbone slightly towards your navel.

- Straighten your right leg. Bend your left knee and place your left foot on the floor in front of your right knee.

- Place your left hand on the floor.

- Inhale deeply through your nose, press your left hand into the floor, squeeze your sitting bones closer to each other and lift your waistline off the floor.

- Exhale, pause, and lift the right leg about 10 cm off the floor.

- Keep breathing deeply and slowly and focus on the inner thigh muscles, holding the stretch for 2 minutes or longer if possible.

- Repeat on the other side.

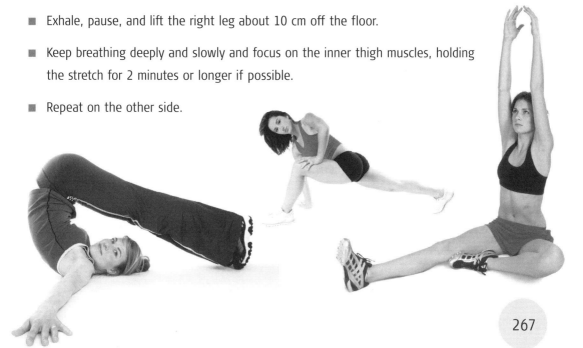

## How did it go?

**Q: If I get started on this deep breathing and stretching, how long will it take before I see an improvement in my cellulite?**

A: It'll take about four weeks, if you do the exercises properly four or five times a week and eat healthily and drink plenty of water to help flush out toxins.

**Q: My cellulite seems to have got worse since I had my baby a few months ago, even though I'm back to my normal weight. Is this hormonal?**

A: It could be a combination of factors, including hormonal shifts, and the fact that exercise regimes often go out of the window post-baby. After pregnancy women are more vulnerable to the pelvis being out of alignment, so the Putkisto method is a good starting point. It also has the big advantage that you can do it at home whenever the baby is asleep – you don't even need to turn up at a class.

Defining idea…

'Those who think they have not time for bodily exercise will sooner or later have to find time for illness.'
EDWARD STANLEY

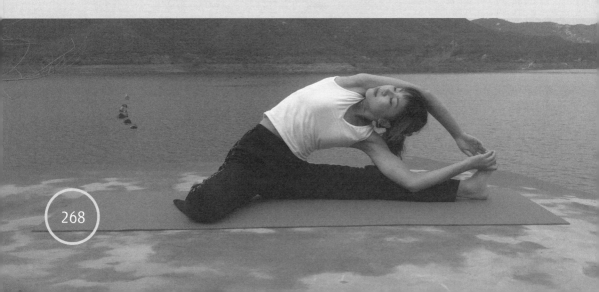

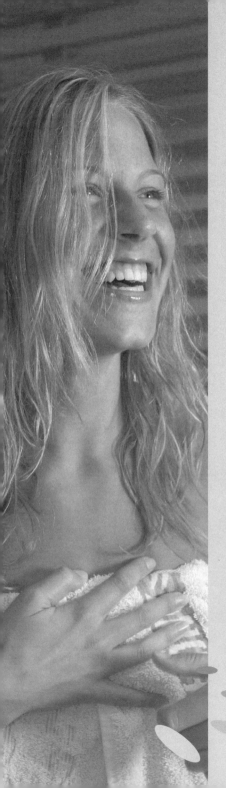

# 48

# Some like it hot

**Saunas and steam rooms open up sweat pores and help eliminate cellulite-causing toxins. So after you've had a dimple-busting workout, get even hotter and sweatier.**

*Relax, purify and de-stress: go somewhere the phone or email can't reach you...saunas are hot, hot hot!*

One of the great things about a session in a sauna is that it's one of the very few places you can genuinely relax. No one will burst through the door asking you for this month's sales figures or demand you tell them where their socks are, 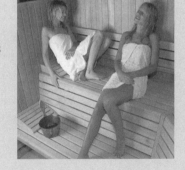 and if they did they'd look pretty silly. And you won't even be able to jot down a shopping list because the paper, if you had any, would go soggy in your sweaty hands.

So make the most of those precious minutes, close your eyes and really let your whole body relax. Even though you only spend a short time (20 minutes or less) in the hot seat, the de-stressing benefits can last long after you've put your clothes back on. And, as we know, over-stressing isn't good for your body, nor is it good for your cellulite. Too much of the stress hormone cortisol can set off a chain of reactions in the body which could have detrimental effects on the digestion and skin, and even lead to weight gain – none of which is going to do your cellulite any good.

The perfect time to head for the sauna or steam room is after some anti-cellulite exercise, whether that's a gym session, jogging or dance class. You'll get the extra benefit of the heat acting as a muscle relaxant, which will help ease any post-workout soreness or stiffness. Not everyone likes the intense heat, but if you do, your sauna session is an added incentive to get down to the health club on those days when your motivation is flagging.

Your body will start to react to the sauna heat as soon as you step through the door. The temperature makes your heart rate increase, boosting your circulation. Your skin may actually get a double boost because the circulatory system sends extra blood flow to the dermis as the skin temperature rises.

> ### Here's an idea for you...
> Never mind that little white towel, appearing nude in the sauna on a regular basis gives you an extra incentive to keep up the good work in your campaign to ditch the crinkly bottom. A hot tip: take off any gold, silver or other metallic necklaces, bracelets or dangly earrings – they'll heat up to such a degree in the sauna that you'll risk burning your skin.

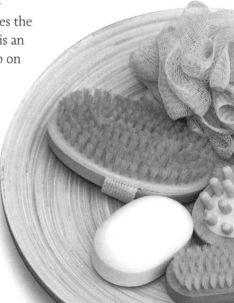

Improved circulation is good for cellulite-prone skin, and it also gives the body's waste disposal system a shove in the right direction, helping to speed up the rate at which toxins are expelled. The heat also opens up the skin's pores, which may further encourage the elimination of toxins.

Hot news in the sauna world are infrared versions, which give off rays of heat from elements positioned inside the wooden cabin. The heat rays target objects (i.e. you sitting in there) instead of heating the air as a traditional sauna does. The rays penetrate deeper into the skin than air heat, making you sweat more, your cardiovascular system work harder, and increasing your metabolism to burn more calories.

By the way, extreme temperatures in any type of sauna have a dramatic impact on your body so be sure to read the health warning notices outside the sauna door, and don't be tempted to stay longer than the recommended time, however de-stressing it is in there.

Because the pores have been opened up and cleansed, post-sauna could also be a good time to massage any anti-cellulite oils or moisturising creams into your dimples. Take your lotions and potions with you so you can slather them on before you get dressed.

*Try another idea...*

**If you like the idea of a sauna, then other spa treatments might appeal to you. Check out IDEA 41, *Getting your sea legs*, for the lowdown on thalassotherapy.**

*Defining idea...*

**'Every time a woman leaves off something she looks better, but every time a man leaves off something he looks worse.'**
WILL ROGERS

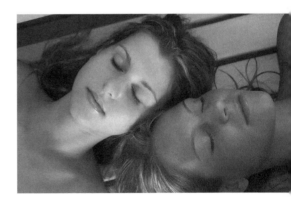

271

Whatever other benefits you get from the 'deep heat' treatment, you leave feeling fantastically cleansed, relaxed and with a definite sense of wellbeing. Your skin feels and looks healthier, and your cheeks (yes, all four of them) are left with a rosy glow, which can make you look years younger.

## How did it go?

**Q: Will regular sauna sessions help me lose weight?**

A: Any weight you lose after a sauna has a lot to do with all that perspiration that's been pouring out of you, and as you need to drink water after a sauna you're likely to regain the weight. The extreme heat of a sauna can increase your metabolic rate so that you burn more calories temporarily, though as you are only in there for 20 minutes this may not make much of a difference. But the new infrared saunas should be a better bet for weight loss as they increase the circulation and metabolism more, helping you burn more calories.

**Q: I'd love to get the benefits of a sauna or steam bath but some weeks I have trouble finding time for a half-hour run, let alone a trip to the health club. Any ideas?**

A: Yes! Turn your bathroom into a mini steam room. Run a deep, hot bath with the ventilator fan switched off and windows and door shut tight so the room gets nice and steamy. Wait for a bit before you get in the bath, though, as water that's too hot can actually make the skin dry. Pour in some scented bath oil, or aromatherapy oil if you have any, fold a small towel to rest your neck on, and lie in the fragrant steaming water with your eyes closed. If you can imagine you're at a luxurious spa, it will help. It may not be quite the same, but you'll still get the therapeutic benefit.

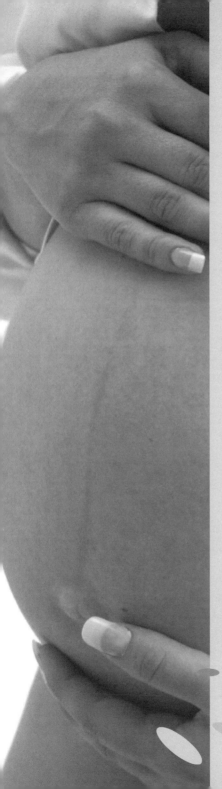

# 49

# Mums, bums and tums

**Extra pounds and hormonal surges during pregnancy often make cellulite worse. Here's how to avoid surplus weight, plus postnatal exercises to firm those wobbly bits.**

Your number one priority when you see that thrilling blue line appear on your

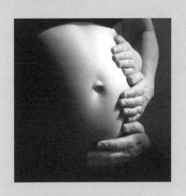

pregnancy test kit is your health, not your cellulite. But stay-healthy strategies will also help keep your thighs as smooth as your baby's bottom...

OK, we've all seen the pictures of skinny celebrities fresh from their birthing pools. These people are generally freaks: it's completely normal to take up to six months to shift the extra weight (and much longer than that for lots of women), and it's also completely normal for cellulite to increase during pregnancy and to still be there afterwards.

The extra oestrogen that's floating around your body during pregnancy means you are more likely to get cellulite. Also, you can't have a healthy pregnancy without storing fat, which will happen automatically to prepare your body for the growing baby and to enable you to produce milk. Then there's the fluid retention some women get when they're pregnant, which has also been blamed for increasing cellulite.

Here's an idea
for you...

**Persevere with breastfeeding. Many new mothers find the weight drops off quickly if they carry on breastfeeding for as long as they can because of the hefty amount of calories breastfeeding uses up. With weight loss goes cellulite loss, and the baby gets the best nutrition possible from your milk – so everyone wins.**

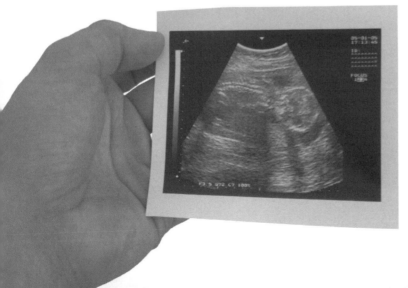

So, expect more cellulite when you're pregnant and you won't be disappointed. It doesn't have to be permanent, though, and there are ways you can have a healthy pregnancy and minimise the amount of orange peel you're going to get.

# How much weight should I put on?

Forget about 'eating for two'. What's important is to eat nutrient-rich foods with lots of fruit and veg and try to ditch any junk food habits and sugary stuff – just the sort of diet that's anti-cellulite, in fact. You need sufficient calories, but if you make being pregnant an excuse to eat a tub of Ben & Jerry's every night you'll find it that much harder to lose the extra post-baby weight – and the cellulite.

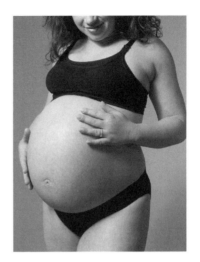

To make it easier to eat more healthily, try these swaps:

- Instead of white bread and pasta, choose wholegrain.

- Swap a plate of biscuits for a plate of sliced fruit.

*Try another idea...*

**If you're at home with your baby, you might find that a good set of stretching exercises will help you regain your shape. IDEA 47, *Bend it, stretch it*, will show you the way.**

- Instead of croissants with your cappuccino, have porridge or muesli with plain yoghurt and blueberries/raspberries.

- Open a packet of nuts (Brazils, cashews, almonds) instead of a packet of crisps.

- Swap fizzy drinks for pure fruit juice or smoothies.

275

After you've spent nine months eating healthier food you're less likely to fall back into bad habits again, which will make it a whole lot easier to get back into shape after your baby is born.

Carry on with regular but gentle exercise throughout your pregnancy: this will help keep cellulite at bay, and will help you to stay fit, healthy and as stress-free as possible – all good for both of you.

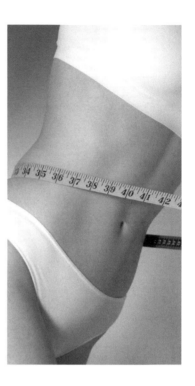

## Post-baby bumps

The first thing to do if you're alarmed by cellulite that's appeared since you've had your baby is: don't panic! Remember that with all that hormonal upheaval it's no wonder your body needs time to settle down.

But you can give the cellulite and wobbly bits a helping hand with simple exercises that you can do any time you've got a spare few minutes. If you're breastfeeding, it's a good idea to exercise straight afterwards so your breasts won't be painfully full of milk (not the ideal time to start jigging around).

For the first few weeks after the birth be careful about exercising, apart from taking your baby out for a walk. Check with your doctor or midwife before you start any exercise to make sure you're ready, particularly if you've had any complications or a Caesarean, and always do some warm-up stretches before you start.

# Lunges for thighs and bottom

This simple exercise will tone up your bottom and thighs. If you've never done lunges before, start with five repeats instead of ten and gradually build up.

**1.** Stand with your feet together and hands on hips.

**2.** Keeping your body upright, take a big step forward with your right leg and lower the left knee towards the floor.

**3.** Step back, and repeat 10 times.

**4.** Do the same with the other leg.

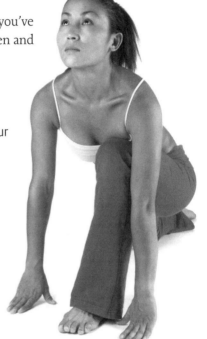

# Tummy trimmers

This is a gentler, but effective, alternative to sit-ups.

**1.** Lie on your back with your knees bent and feet flat on the floor.

**2.** Slide your feet as far forward as you can while still keeping them flat on the floor.

**3.** With your head and shoulders raised off the floor, stretch your arms by your sides a few inches off the floor, with fingers pointing towards your feet.

**4.** Alternately stretch your right hand towards your right toes, then left hand towards left toes, moving your upper body from side to side.

**5.** Count 20 stretches (10 each side) then rest before doing another set. Aim to do three sets.

## How did it go?

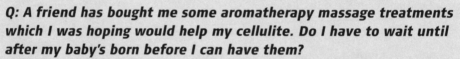

**Q: I'm only three months pregnant but I've already put on 2 kilos. Is this normal?**

A: Yes – 2 kg during the first trimester is spot on. Although the baby doesn't weigh anything like 2 kg at this stage, your body needs to lay down fat deposits. Some women will gain more weight during these early stages, especially if they are prone to fluid retention, others less if they are throwing up and have lost their appetite due to morning sickness.

**Q: A friend has bought me some aromatherapy massage treatments which I was hoping would help my cellulite. Do I have to wait until after my baby's born before I can have them?**

A: Some cellulite treatments are best avoided while you're pregnant, so always tell any therapist you are seeing as soon as you know you are expecting. Aromatherapy oils can be very powerful and some are not recommended during pregnancy. But just think how lovely those pampering treatments will be after the birth! (By the way, some aromatherapy oils are also good for stretch marks.)

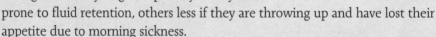

Defining idea...
*'With what price we pay for the glory of motherhood.'*
ISADORA DUNCAN

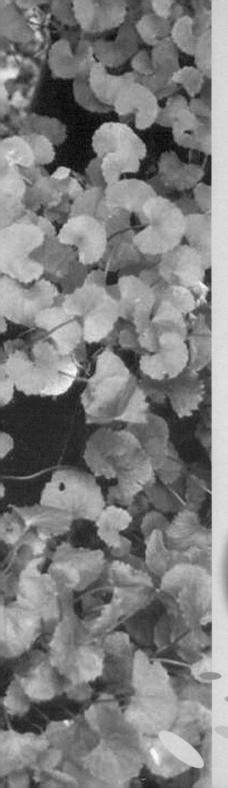

## 50

# Grass roots

**Clinical trials show that the herb gotu kola could reduce your cellulite by strengthening connective tissue and increasing circulation.**

It sounds wacky, but this is one herbal remedy that's got some science behind it.

279

One thing all the experts who've devoted years to studying cellulite agree on is this: the reason it looks unpleasantly like cottage cheese is because fat is protruding through the honeycomb of 'connective' tissue that is supposed to keep it in place. Think of flabby thighs in a pair of fishnet stockings that are a size too small (if you dare). If we could strengthen these connective tissues, so that they do their job properly and keep the fat where it should be, then we would be taking a big step towards solving the cellulite problem.

That's where this weird-sounding herb comes in. Because it's been used for thousands of years in folk medicine (no fly-by-night fad, this), scientists have been intrigued to find out more about it, so there's been quite a bit of research. Without going into incomprehensible scientific detail, a lot of the studies suggest the herb's abilities include stimulating the body's production of substances that strengthen those connective tissues. You get the connection?

> Here's an idea for you...
>
> If you've bought some gotu kola but haven't got round to trying it yet, get it out of the cupboard. You might find it works on more than just your cellulite. It has a long history of treating various ailments. It's even said to improve memory, help stave off senility and ageing and increase intelligence, so you may get more benefits than you bargained for.

Another thing that comes up again and again in research documents is that gotu kola can improve circulation and blood flow, which is why it has long been used to help heal skin diseases. It has also been used to treat varicose veins and other problems caused by reduced blood flow, with excellent results. In discussions with both beauty experts and medical professionals, improving the circulation comes up regularly as a key to reducing cellulite. Still more studies show that it could help by stimulating the lymph system to get rid of excess fluids – the dreaded water retention that makes cellulite look worse.

And there's more. Gotu kola is one of very few herbs that has been investigated with a clinical trial specifically for its effect on cellulite. Sixty-five women with cellulite who had already tried various ways of reducing it without success were given gotu kola for a period of three months. At the end of the experiment, over three-quarters of the women noticed a difference in their cellulite, with 58% reporting that the results were 'very good' and 20% saying the improvement was 'satisfactory'.

Want to know more about this 'magic' plant? It's a type of tropical creeper, and if you're of a scientific disposition and want to look it up, here's a bit of help. Its Latin name is *Centella asiatica*, and you'll sometimes find it spelt gota kola instead of gotu. Got it? Good, and have fun among the boffins.

*Try another idea...*

**It's easy to do, takes only seconds, and it's free! Why the simple act of drinking a glass of water is one of the best things you can do for your body – and your cellulite. Go straight to IDEA 13, *Still waters*.**

*Defining idea...*

**'The method of nature: who could ever analyse it?'**
RALPH WALDO EMERSON

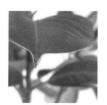 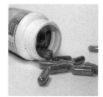 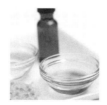 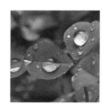

# How do you take it?

■ You can find gotu kola in supplement form in pharmacies and health food stores. The recommendation for cellulite is to take 30 mg three times a day, which herbalists reckon is sufficient to strengthen the connective tissue and keep skin smooth.

■ The dried herb can be used to make a tea which you can drink several times a day. You can buy it from health shops and herbalists who will be able to give you advice on how much to use.

■ If the only tea you like is a nice brown colour and goes with biscuits, you can buy gotu kola in tincture form and squeeze a few drops into a drink.

■ Oil and creams containing gotu kola are used to massage into the body to rehydrate the skin. You can order oil via the internet, plus some salons use oil or creams as part of their anti-cellulite treatments.

As with so many cellulite-shifting methods, think of this herb as part of an overall regime rather than a solution in itself. So it goes without saying (but we'll say it anyway) that it would be a waste of time and money to swallow gotu kola supplements while living the life of a dehydrated, junk food-munching couch potato (which we're sure you're not).

PS: If you are taking any kind of medication, it's better to clear it with your doctor before you start on any herbal remedies or supplements, and it's safer to avoid gotu kola if you're pregnant.

# How did it go?

**Q: All these different ways of taking this herb have got me confused. I don't know whether to swallow a capsule, make it into a tea or rub it on my bottom. What do you suggest?**

A: Taking it in its purest form, so that it's not diluted with other ingredients, is probably the best. So try buying the dried herbs and making a tea. There's no reason why you can't follow a two-pronged approach and drink tea and rub a lotion or oil into your skin, or take supplements and use a cream. Just remember not to drink the lotion and rub the tea into your thighs.

**Q: Can I grow gotu kola in the herb patch in my garden then, so I've got a readymade supply?**

A: Probably not, unless you happen to live on the edge of a marsh in the tropics. But it's becoming more popular, so you should be able to find it in a herbalist's or health food store.

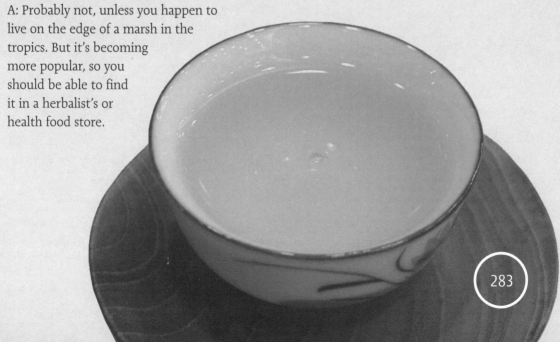

Defining idea...
'The system of nature, of which man is a part, tends to be self-balancing.'
ISAAC ASIMOV

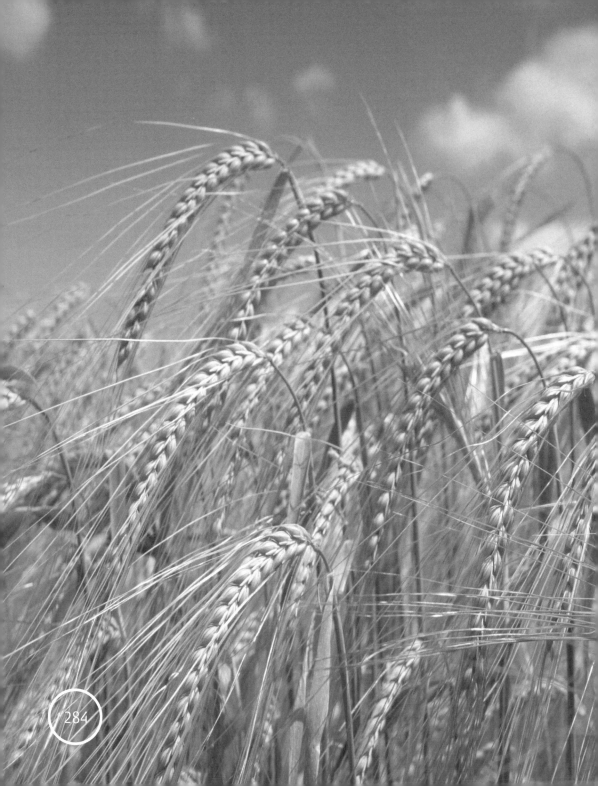

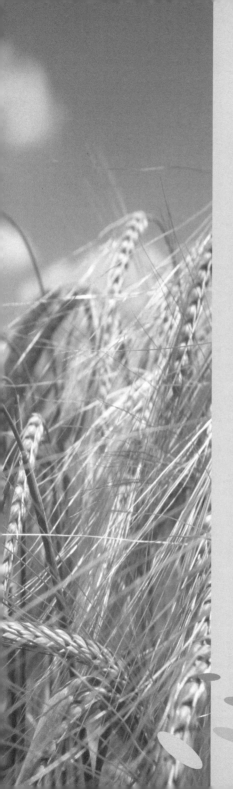

# 51

# The winds of change

**Bloating is not the only side-effect of wheat intolerance; it may also make cellulite worse. Try our sensible food swaps.**

Wheat intolerance may sound like one of those 'fashionable' complaints, but it's no joke if your stomach feels like you've swallowed a football every time you eat a bowl of pasta. And doing something about it could have other benefits too.

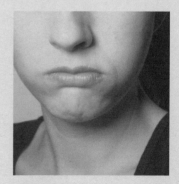

First things first: wheat intolerance is different to wheat allergy. In fact, very few people have a full-blown allergy to wheat, but a much larger group have varying degrees of sensitivity to it – an intolerance. Wheat intolerance is not as extreme as an allergy, but it can give you that uncomfortable, bloated feeling after meals containing wheat. Worse, it can give you quite bad stomach pains. Headaches can be a symptom, as can fluid retention – which can also contribute to cellulite.

Problems with your digestive system mean that your body isn't working as efficiently as it should be, and poor digestion can inhibit absorption of vitamins and minerals. It may also mean that the elimination of toxins isn't exactly going to plan – another problem linked to cellulite. Added to this, some cellulite-watching experts believe that bloating caused by excess gas in the system – from food that hasn't been broken down properly – impairs another of the body's waste disposal methods, the lymph system. Again, poor lymphatic drainage is linked to cellulite.

Much of the Western diet is based on wheat and it's what we've grown to love: bread, pasta, pastry, cakes, biscuits, pizza... Wheat is also hidden in countless manufactured foods, from

Here's an idea for you...

**The first thing to do, if you are experiencing discomfort after eating certain foods, is to keep a food diary for two weeks and write down everything you eat and any symptoms. The first person to show this to is your GP, who will decide whether to refer you to a dietician for further investigation.**

ready-to-cook dinners to sauces, salad dressings, crisps and other snacks. With all this lot, most of us are getting wheat several times a day, and it's too much for some of us.

The good news is that there are ever-increasing options for the wheat avoider and you don't even have to root about in health shops – the bigger supermarkets now have whole sections of wheat-free goodies. And many wheat-sensitive people find once they have cut back and reduced or eliminated their uncomfortable symptoms, they can tolerate small amounts of wheat.

So if you suffer from bloating and stomach pain or discomfort after meals, it's worth assessing how much wheat you've just eaten. But, as with any health problem, see a doctor first in case there is another reason for the symptoms.
If she gives you the all-clear, then go ahead – but make sure you have enough carbohydrates and fibre in your diet to stay healthy.
Try the following food swaps.

*Try another idea...*
**Hold the front page! Research is going on all the time to find new and better ways of reducing cellulite. Get ahead of the pack – for a sneak preview of the very latest discoveries go straight to IDEA 27, *The next big thing?***

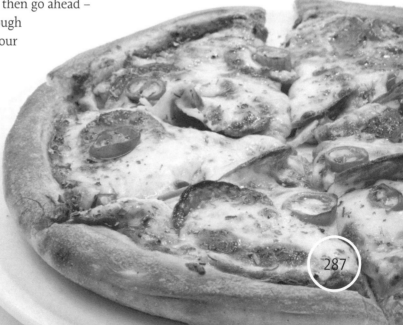

# Swap shop

### Bread
Replace bread with oatcakes (yummy with cheese), rice cakes, good old Ryvita or taco shells. Try wheat-free breads, made from rice flour or rye flour.

### Breakfast cereals
If you're a toast and cereals kind of girl, you might be left wondering what you're going to have for breakfast, since standard loaves contain wheat and so do most cereals. Try switching to corn- or rice-based cereals such as cornflakes, and look out for wheat-free muesli. But a great breakfast is porridge (oats, not wheat), even the instant variety which you can do in the microwave as quick as a flash. Add some berries and plain yoghurt or crème fraiche and you have a delicious breakfast that will keep your energy levels up until lunchtime.

Or why not base your breakfast around fruit and yoghurt. Plain yoghurt poured over chopped banana (great for morning energy), and berries such as strawberries, blueberries and raspberries (full of healthy antioxidants), gives you a good start to the day.

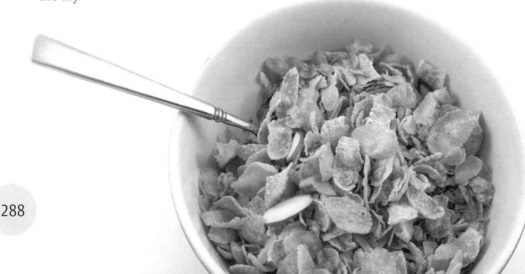

## Lunchtime sandwiches

Wheat-free can be tricky if you're used to grabbing a sandwich for lunch. But again, this could be the trigger to finding a healthier alternative. Salad and soup is a good alternative, and many sandwich shops also offer a tasty soup of the day. Pick one with loads of veg in it, followed by a favourite salad including protein (such as tuna, prawn, chicken), then a piece of fruit and you're well on your way to your five portions of fruit and veg a day. And ring the changes with rice-based sushi, another healthy alternative to sandwiches.

> ### Defining idea...
> **'If I'd known I was gonna live this long, I'd have taken better care of myself.'**
> EUBIE BLAKE, veteran jazz pianist

## Pasta

Love pasta? No problem, there are now lots of different wheat-free pasta products on the market. Try pasta made from rice or corn, or choose rice or rice noodles instead.

## Cakes/biscuits

Reach for the fruit bowl instead of the biscuit tin – keep it stocked with your favourites. OK, OK, it's not the same, but if you're craving something sweet try the sweeter fruits such as grapes, bananas or apricots. If you really can't hack it without something gooey, go for oatcakes with low-sugar jam. Or buy biscuits made with oats not wheat – but remember, sugar-laden biscuits of any type are best avoided if you're serious about getting rid of cellulite.

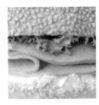 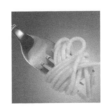 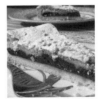

## How did it go?

**Q: I love bread but that dark rye bread just isn't the same, is it? Any other ideas?**

A: The very dark rye bread does have a strong flavour and is a bit of an acquired taste, but the lighter-coloured ones are different. Try some of the others such as pumpernickel – keep sampling until you find one you like! Or better still, make it yourself.

**Q: So how can buckwheat be OK if you're wheat intolerant?**

A: Because it's not wheat, that's why. Confused? Who can blame you. Buckwheat is another type of grain altogether. You can get buckwheat flour, noodles and even buckwheat pancake mix, so if you spot any of these you can put them straight in your shopping basket. Happy label-reading!

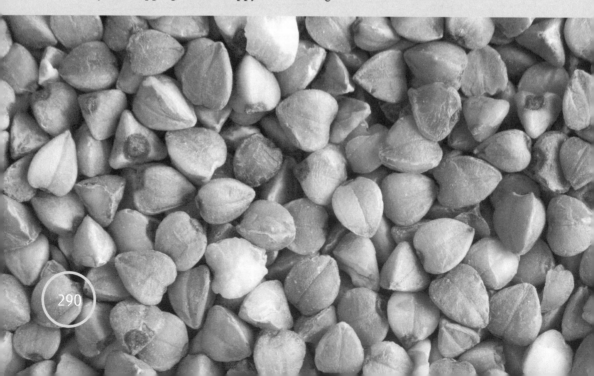

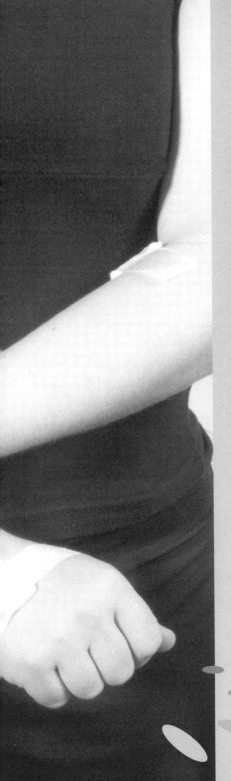

# 52

# Getting plastered

**Those clever scientists! Now they've given us cellulite-busting patches that you stick on your bottom and thighs, from where they send skin-improving minerals direct to your trouble spots. Whatever next?**

Nicotine patches, HRT patches, patches for bags under your eyes, even patches to cure hangovers...there seems to be a stick-on solution for just about everything now — and that includes cellulite.

Like nicotine patches, the ingredients in an anti-cellulite patch are designed to be slowly absorbed into the skin over a certain period, whether for a few hours or a whole day and night. The patches often come in boxes of a week's or a month's supply, with the essential ingredients in a liquid or gel form inside the patch. A peel-off adhesive strip allows you to stick them on your worst-offending areas, then you just leave them there to do their job, while you carry on doing whatever you want.

The patches vary in size and, frankly, some of them look too small to be able to do anything for all that dimply flesh. But the theory is that the ingredients spread outwards to treat an area several times bigger than the patch itself – which may be a relief for those of us with family-sized crinkly bottoms.

So what's in these patches? One of the main ingredients is caffeine. Caffeine crops up in other cellulite-busting treatments, based on laboratory experiments which have shown its ability to boost cell metabolism, plus the knowledge that it can be absorbed through the skin.

Other ingredients in the patches are usually a cocktail of mineral, herbal or seaweed extracts aimed at either draining fluid from the tissues in the area, boosting the skin's micro-circulation or improving skin texture. Many of the ingredients are

> *Here's an idea for you...*
>
> **Improving your posture can work wonders for your cellulite – instantly. Slouching makes all your saggy bits look, well, saggier, but drawing yourself up to your full height makes your skin tauter and smoothes out some of the crinkles, especially on your stomach. Standing upright with your head held high also automatically gives you more confidence in yourself and how you look. So find the nearest mirror and practise giving yourself an instant 'lift'. Magic!**

similar to the ones in anti-cellulite creams – the idea is that they are absorbed by the skin more easily via patches. Ingredients may be activated by body heat, the heat apparently helping the absorption. Also, some patches contain substances that make them heat up when they're next to the skin – a bit like the hand warmers you put in your ski gloves – giving you 'hot legs' or even a 'hot bot' – you have been warned (or is that 'warmed'?)

*Try another idea...*
**What can having green goo that smells of the sea smothered all over you, then being wrapped in clingfilm, do for your cellulite? Find out by turning to IDEA 9, *The green goddess*.**

Some pretty serious health complaints are now being treated using skin patches, including prostate problems in men, which shows the potential power of 'patch therapy'. But having said that, so far the results from cellulite patch-wearers are, shall we say, 'patchy'. So what can anyone expect from them?

We've taken into account the opinions of several cellulite-plagued lovelies on this one. Their experiences vary widely, from 'couldn't see any difference' to 'my skin looked smoother and felt firmer'.

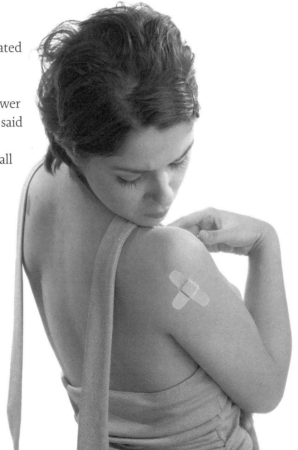

Others who measured their thighs before wearing patches for around a month have reported a loss of as much as 4 cm from their thigh circumference and smoother-looking skin. However, they were also following other anti-cellulite ideas such as body brushing, drinking more water and exercising, so it's hard to tell which method was working for them.

There have also been some reports of patches causing a burning sensation to the skin, so proceed (or not) with caution is the message, particularly if tempted to order over the internet. As with any product, it's safer to buy from established brand names than those you've never heard of, and always follow manufacturer's instructions to the letter. If it says don't wear them for more than eight hours or more than twice a week, don't.

It may be that, like some of the creams, the role of patches is to improve the appearance of the skin that covers the cellulite – so that it looks firmer and smoother – rather than affect the underlying cellulite itself. And it could be easier to judge the results, even if temporary, on a small area, like dimply fat over the knees.

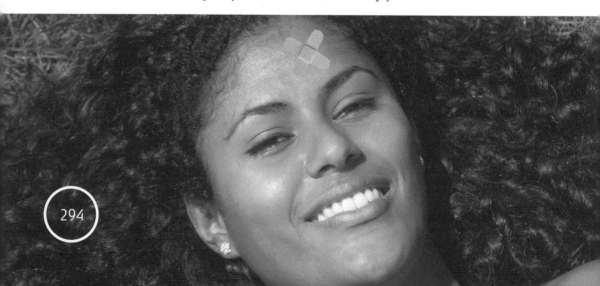

## How did it go?

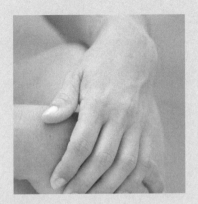

**Q: I don't fancy wearing patches with my best sexy lingerie when I'm hoping for a night of romance. Would it make any difference if I took them off for a while?**

A: Good point, sticking on anti-cellulite patches might not put you in the sexiest of moods, even if he never notices them. But if you've started wearing them, taking them off would be a waste of time and money. So if you want to try them, check out the manufacturer's instructions first and choose ones you don't have to wear for 24 hours. Some recommend eight hours, so you could wear them during the day under clothes.

**Q: My cellulite covers an area the size of Peru (well almost) – all over my bottom, thighs and backs of my legs – I admit I'm about 10 kg overweight. Am I going to have to use dozens of patches?**

A: Hmm. Sounds as if you'll be better off sticking something else on your lower half – like cycling shorts, or maybe just jeans and a pair of sturdy walking boots and taking yourself off for some good old-fashioned exercise instead. It's always better to shift excess weight first if you're serious about reducing cellulite, and brisk walking and cycling (and running, but be careful if you haven't done much exercise lately) burns calories, tones the muscles, boosts the circulation and helps improve cellulite anyway – a triple whammy. And a blast of exercise in the fresh air will get the endorphins – the body's 'feel-good' chemicals – going too, helping you to stay motivated. Now where did you put those trainers?

> *Defining idea...*
> **'Taking joy in living is a woman's best cosmetic.'**
> ROSALIND RUSSELL

# The end...

Or is it a new beginning? We hope that the ideas in this book will have inspired you to try some new things to ditch your dimples for good. You've swapped your coffee for water, started walking or jogging more and are keeping up the regular body brushing. Next time you go to the beach you'll be disrobing with confidence.

So why not let *us* know all about it? Tell us how you got on. What did it for you – what really made a difference to your thighs or bottom? Maybe you've got some tips of your own you want to share (see next page if so). And if you liked this book you may find we have even more brilliant ideas that could change other areas of your life for the better.

You'll find the Infinite Ideas crew waiting for you online at www.infideas.com.

Or if you prefer to write, then send your letters to:

*Cellulite solutions*
The Infinite Ideas Company Ltd
36 St Giles, Oxford OX1 3LD, United Kingdom

We want to know what you think, because we're all working on making our lives better too. Give us your feedback and you could win a copy of another *52 Brilliant Ideas* book of your choice. Or maybe get a crack at writing your own.

Good luck. Be brilliant.

# Offer one

## CASH IN YOUR IDEAS

We hope you enjoy this book. We hope it inspires, amuses, educates and entertains you. But we don't assume that you're a novice, or that this is the first book that you've bought on the subject. You've got ideas of your own. Maybe our authors have missed an idea that you use successfully. If so, why not send it to yourauthormissedatrick@infideas.com, and if we like it we'll post it on our bulletin board. Better still, if your idea makes it into print we'll send you four books of your choice or the cash equivalent. You'll be fully credited so that everyone knows you've had another Brilliant Idea.

# Offer two

## HOW COULD YOU REFUSE?

Amazing discounts on bulk quantities of Infinite Ideas books are available to corporations, professional associations and other organisations.

For details call us on:
+44 (0)1865 514888
Fax: +44 (0)1865 514777
or e-mail: info@infideas.com

# Where it's at...

# CHAMPNEYS

### HEALTH RESORTS

**All 'Cellulite solutions' readers can enjoy 15% off ALL standard tariff packages at Champneys until end of December 2006 and 10% off ALL cellulite solution treatments!**

Champneys provides a selection of premier health resorts across the United Kingdom offering relaxing treatments, healthy cuisine, exceptional spa facilities and friendly service. A family run business, Champneys prides itself on offering exceptional standards in beauty, fitness, nutrition and holistic wellbeing. Boasting the latest spa technologies complemented by friendly and amenable staff Champneys has become a chain of resorts unrivalled in luxury and beauty.

Each health resort is unique with its own distinct personality. The resorts cater for everyone, and are ideal to visit on your own, with friends or as a couple. Choose from the original and recently refurbished Champneys Tring in Hertfordshire, the modern Springs in Leicestershire, the enchanting Forest Mere in Hampshire or Henlow in Bedfordshire.

You can pamper and relax your senses with their exclusive range of beauty and complementary therapies. With over 100 treatments available, therapists use only the finest products from Babor, Elemis and their own Champneys Spa Collection.

Champneys has pioneered the way in health, bringing the concept of holistic health – 'mind, body and soul' – into the public awareness, and now you can experience all it has to offer at a special discounted rate until December 2006.

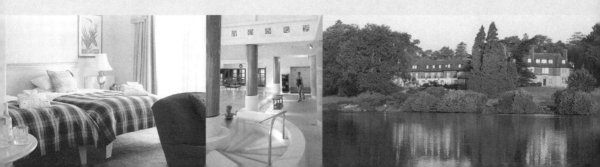

# Enjoy an exclusive 10% discount

In partnership with *Cellulite solutions* Champneys are offering YOU the chance to take advantage of the following discounts when booking at any UK Champneys health resort during 2006.

**15% off any standard tariff booking made before December 2006!**
Bookings can be made via telephone through the Champneys reservation team on **08703 300 300**; please remember to quote the promotional code *'Champneys52'* when booking to receive your discount.
*All Champneys packages include accommodation, all meals and unlimited use of facilities.*

**10% off any of the following specialist cellulite treatments before December 2006!**
All treatments must be booked 2–3 weeks in advance by completing the pre-booking treatment form sent to you with your confirmation. Please note that treatments cannot be booked via telephone and must be booked in writing. Treatments can only be booked within a Champneys package.
*Please remember to quote 'Champneys 52' when booking to qualify for your discount.*

**Champneys Hip and Thigh Detoxifier** – *25 minutes* (Usual price £34.95)
This localised treatment specifically targets areas that are prone to cellulite. Body brushing and exfoliating techniques are combined with a drainage massage resulting in legs feeling firm, smooth and toned!

**Champneys Citrus Body Glow** – *25 minutes* (Usual price £34.95)
Experience an invigorating full body scrub and citrus body oil application, which will stimulate dull, lifeless skin leaving your body feeling smooth and conditioned.

**Babor Modellage** – *55 minutes* (Usual price £55.95)
An anti cellulite/slimming treatment using algae and thermal clay to treat a specific problem area. The result is firm contours and smooth skin.

# CHAMPNEYS
### HEALTH RESORTS

**Elemis Fennel Cleansing Cellulite and Colon Therapy** - *55 minutes* (Usual price £59.95)
This treatment works at the deepest levels to flush and cleanse the system. A detoxifying fennel and birch body mask is applied to hips and thighs and followed by a specialised drainage massage to smooth the appearance of the skin. In addition, cleansing of the colon through abdominal massage and reflexology continues the purification of the body.

**Champneys Complete Wax Experience** - *55 minutes* (Usual price £49.95)
Total indulgence: the body will be relaxed, detoxified and the skin left soft and smooth. To start the body is exfoliated to remove dead skin cells, followed by a full body application of warm whisked soft paraffin wax. You will be left to relax and after the wax is gently peeled away the therapist will apply selected body oils or creams.

**Champneys Body Gold** - *55 minutes* (Usual price £49.95)
This treatment was originally developed for hospitals to treat various lymphatic disorders. This now involves specially designed garments that recreate the effleurage effect.The treatment helps to break down cellulite, remove toxins and improve skin tone. The Body Gold can also benefit conditions such as varicose veins, sports injuries and lymphoedema. It is localised for the leg area.

Exercise is obviously a key factor in the treatment of cellulite and we have experts at Champneys who are available to advise our guests on specific exercise regimes to suit their individual requirements.

# Competition

**Would you like to experience the relaxation and luxury of a Champneys health resort?**

All *Cellulite solutions* readers have the chance of winning a Champneys all-inclusive overnight break for two, including complimentary meals, unlimited use of all facilities and a Champneys Body Massage and Relaxing Facial per person.

To be in with a chance of winning this fantastic Champneys prize, just answer the following question using the information provided:

Which Champneys cellulite treatment uses algae and thermal clay? Is it:

(a) Champneys Citrus Body Glow
(b) Champneys Hip and Thigh Detoxifier
(c) Champneys Babor Modellage

Please send answers to **champneys@infideas.com** or post your answer to 'Champneys Cellulite Competition', Infinite Ideas, 36 St Giles, Oxford OX1 3LD, stating your name, address and a contact telephone number.

The closing date for entries is 30 September 2006. Offer open to UK residents only. The winner will be picked at random and notified via telephone. This prize can be claimed within 1 year from the closing date. Terms and conditions apply, see www.infideas.com

*We never give details to third parties nor will we bombard you with lots of junk mail!*

Good Luck!

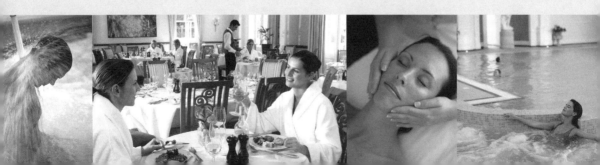